EVERYDAY
HEALTH
HINTS

The Prevention Total Health System®

EVERYDAY HEALTH HINTS

by the Editors of
Prevention® Magazine

 Rodale Press, Emmaus, Pennsylvania

Library of Congress Cataloging in Publication Data

Main entry under title:

Everyday health hints.

(The Prevention total health system)
Includes index.
1. Self-care, Health. 2. Health behavior.
3. Medicine, Popular. 4. Health. I. Prevention.
II. Series.
RA776.95.E94   1985   613   84-22883

ISBN 0-87857-538-3   hardcover
    4 6 8 10 9 7 5 3   hardcover

NOTICE

The Prevention Total Health System®

Series Editors: William Gottlieb, Mark Bricklin
Everyday Health Hints Editor: Jan Bresnick
Writers: Stephen Williams (Chapters 1, 4); Marian Wolbers (Chapter 2), with Jean Sherman; Susan DeMark (Chapter 3); Neal Fandek (Chapters 5, 9); Susan DeMark, Sharon Faelten (Chapter 6); Denise Foley (Chapter 7); Neal Fandek, Ed Weiner (Chapter 8)
Research Chief: Carol Baldwin
Associate Research Chiefs, Prevention Health Books: Susan Nastasee, Christy Kohler
Assistant Research Chief, Prevention Health Books: Holly Clemson
Researchers: Freda Christie, Tawna Clelan, Anne Oplinger, Carole Rapp, Jan Eickmeier, David Palmer, Jill Polk
Copy Editor: Jane Sherman
Copy Coordinator: Joann Williams
Series Art Director: Jerry O'Brien
Art Production Manager: Jane C. Knutila
Designers: Lynn Foulk, Alison Lee
Illustrators: Bascove, Susan M. Blubaugh, Mary Anne Shea, Elwood H. Smith, Chris Spollen, Wendy Wray
Associate Designer: John Pepper
Project Assistant: Lisa Gatti
Director of Photography: T. L. Gettings
Photo Editor: Margaret Skrovanek
Staff Photographers: Angelo M. Caggiano, Mitchell T. Mandel, Alison Miksch, Margaret Skrovanek, Christie C. Tito
Photographic Stylists: Renee R. Keith, J. C. Vera
Photo Researcher: Donna Lewis
Production Manager: Jacob V. Lichty
Production Coordinator: Barbara A. Herman
Composite Typesetter: Brenda J. Kline
Production Administrator: Eileen Bauder
Office Personnel: Susan K. Lagler, Roberta Mulliner, Carol Petrakovich, Cindy Harig, Marge Kresley, Connie Shollenberger, Diana Gottshall

Rodale Books, Inc.
Publisher: Richard M. Huttner
Senior Managing Editor: William H. Hylton
Copy Manager: Ann Snyder
Art Director: Karen A. Schell
Director of Marketing: Pat Corpora
Business Manager: Ellen J. Greene

Rodale Press, Inc.
Chairman of the Board: Robert Rodale
President: Robert Teufel
Executive Vice President: Marshall Ackerman
Group Vice Presidents: Sanford Beldon
                                     Mark Bricklin
Senior Vice President: John Haberern
Vice Presidents: John Griffin
                         Richard M. Huttner
                         James C. McCullagh
                         David Widenmyer
Secretary: Anna Rodale

Contents

Preface

Better Health Begins at Home

People today are remarkably healthy, if you think about it. The epidemics of deadly influenza, polio and all the rest have pretty much been tamed. The terrible industrial accidents that used to be so common a generation or two ago have been reduced dramatically. The heart disease rate is going down, and so is the incidence of stroke. We're quitting the butts, buckling up and belting less booze.

So the time is right to pause for a moment or two and consider the challenge of small things. The health *nuisances.* The irritations and aches, the itches and ouches of everyday living.

Knowing how to deal with these nuisances may not save your life, but it *can* save you from moments that are definitely not worth being alive for, and from thinking what a darn fool you are when your picnic guest is stung by a bee and you don't know whether to put barbecue sauce on it or call the MedEvac chopper.

Preparing material for *Everyday Health Hints* and other books has helped me through many panicky moments.

The time I slammed the car door on my index finger was a good example. Instead of watching it turn black like a hot dog burning on a grill, I swung into my junior paramedic act. I filled a bucket with ice cubes, added some water and plunged my whole hand in. After a minute, I took my hand out, held it over my head and then squeezed the smashed tip of my finger with my other hand. After about ten repetitions of this routine, my finger wasn't black and blue, bleeding or even particularly painful, and even my poor fingernail lived to tell the story.

I've eased some wicked sunburns simply by splashing vinegar on the affected area, repeating every 5 or 10 minutes.

I've short-circuited headaches by pressing the temples and the back of the skull with my fingertips.

On the trail, I've stopped small blisters on my feet from turning into mushroom caps by applying moleskin at the first instant of ouchness.

In the plane, I've prevented the earaches I used to get by practicing the modified Valsalva maneuver (see page 22).

And, on the job, I've learned that putting a molded foam rubber cushion on the chair that I'm sitting in as I write these words will save me from having a backache when I stand up.

The practical aspects of *Everyday Health Hints* are a true cornucopia of coping measures, but I think they're only half the story. There's a kind of philosophical side, too. I find it somehow bracing to know that I can handle a lot of life's little bumps and boo-boos. Don't we already depend on experts for enough things? Just for the sake of balance, shouldn't we begin to bone up on a body of knowledge so useful to our personal well-being?

If you believe we should, you will find *Everyday Health Hints* to be an especially enjoyable part of The Prevention Total Health System.®

Executive Editor, **Prevention**® Magazine

1

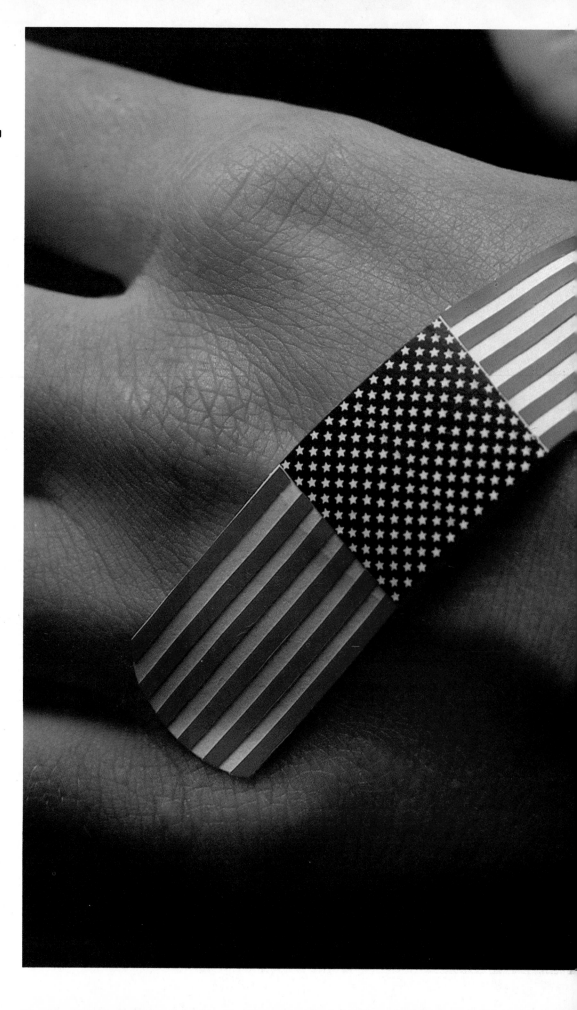

The Self-Care Revolution

Armed with information, medical consumers can go a long way toward becoming independently healthy.

You wake up damp on sweat-soaked sheets, frightened because you are ill but don't know the cause. You touch your forehead; it's hot and moist, as though you had just stepped out of the bath. You wonder, "How serious is it?"

Someone calls the doctor for you, because your throat is sore and it hurts to talk. Later, after sitting in the waiting room for 40 minutes, you hear your doctor's $35 diagnosis: "It's a bug that's going around. Drink lots of fluids, stay warm and get plenty of rest."

Your son smells pudding boiling on the stove, rushes into the kitchen from the living room and catches you blind-sided as you fill the dessert cups. The hot pot falls from your hand, scattering scalding pudding along your son's arm. He's in such pain that you carry him to the car and rush to the emergency room. "He'll be all right," says the doctor, "but you could have saved the little guy a lot of hurt if you'd just stuck the arm in cold water before bringing him in."

If neither of these scenarios is very comforting, consider this one:

You get home from a hard day at work feeling fatigued, light-headed and hoarse. You fix a cup of herb tea and look up your symptoms in the easy-to-read medical guide your doctor suggested. Page 59 tells you to take your temperature, drink plenty of fluids and rest until morning. You wake up early, still feeling ill, and take your own throat culture with a kit your doctor gave you on your last visit. Your daughter drops off the culture at a nearby laboratory and that afternoon you receive a call saying your test is negative. The book advises you on what to eat and says to get plenty of rest—there's nothing else to do but wait out the illness. Three days later the symptoms are gone and you haven't had to visit your doctor or take any medication. You've safely treated yourself and you feel good about it.

This scenario is what self-care is all about: active participation in your own medical care. Self-care is the culmination of the belief that you have the greatest stake in your own health.

A NATURAL RESPONSE TO ILLNESS

You probably practice some form of self-care now without even realizing it. It's estimated that for every symptom of illness doctors see, seven more go unreported, taken care of at home with the aid of family and friends. Each time you clean and bandage a cut, you are practicing self-care. "The fact is," says Lowell Levin, Ed.D., M.P.H., of the Yale University School of Medicine, "if people stopped doing self-care, they probably wouldn't survive until Friday."

But self-care can go beyond

treating simple cuts and bruises; it can deal with problems like flu, back pain or insomnia. It's a way of taking charge of your life. "The basic principle of self-care," says Tom Ferguson, M.D., editor of *Medical Self-Care* magazine, "is that you rely more on yourself. You realize that doctors and other health professionals—whether they offer traditional or alternative medicine— are useful resources, but no one has the whole answer. You are the only one who carries total responsibility for yourself, and you can manage your health care better than anyone else."

Modern self-care encompasses every available resource that can reasonably help you manage your health, from simple kits that allow you to test yourself at home for pregnancy or high blood pressure to pamphlets and self-help books like this one.

That the trend toward self-care is changing the face of medical treatment in America can't be doubted. As people become more knowledgeable about self-testing with computers and other tools, "the doctor will become more a medical technician working with the consumer/patient than a godlike

The cost of living—healthy living—jumps higher and higher, while the average person's ability to pay drops. While you may think that health-care price hikes affect only your insurance company, not you, the fact is you ultimately pay the bill in higher taxes and insurance premiums. The solution: self-care. "Healthy habits could save people and business a substantial amount of money," says one economist.

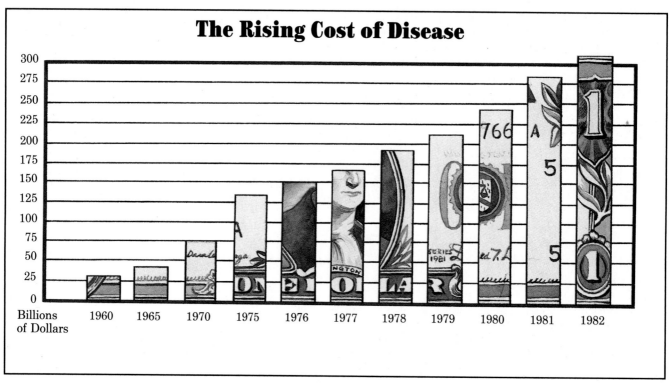

The Rising Cost of Disease

Billions of Dollars: 1960, 1965, 1970, 1975, 1976, 1977, 1978, 1979, 1980, 1981, 1982

figure working on the consumer," says Charles Inlander, executive director of the People's Medical Society, an organization devoted to consumer participation.

Doctors see the resulting change in attitude as remarkable: "Five or six years ago the doctor-patient relationship reached an all-time low, but there have been great improvements since then. Doctors used to see themselves as mythical types, and people bought it. But no more," says one family doctor.

According to another, "Younger doctors are finally beginning to acknowledge the importance of self-care and patient education."

Leonard Borman, Ph.D., president of The Self-Help Center of Chicago, concurs: "I find a new sympathy among M.D.'s to learn about self-help, and there is now proof that self-help works. It has become a major movement; it's not like the hula hoop, because it won't go away. Self-help meets people's needs."

But how safe is self-care? "There's no such thing as absolute safety," says Dr. Levin. "In my judgment, the hazards of quick-fix professional service far outweigh any hazards that might be involved in self-care. I can only say that, for minor illnesses and injuries, if people are motivated and have some knowledge, skill and access to tools, they do very well most of the time. Generally, people are pretty sensible about when they really need a professional."

Countless examples of self-care in action back up Dr. Levin's statement. Here are a few.

SOLVING BACK PROBLEMS

"Oh, my aching back," is the refrain of countless commercials for pain-killers and lotions that promise relief from back pain. Judging from the continuing stream of televised complaints, however, few of these products offer more than temporary, minor relief. Fortunately, we needn't rely on them. There *is* a way to get lasting, effective and cost-free relief from back pain at home.

The Center for Pain Studies at

Doctors' Strike: A Matter of Life, Not Death

What if all the doctors in America suddenly ascended to that great golf course in the sky, leaving their earthly practices behind? "It would be disastrous," you might say. "How would we survive?"

Pretty well, probably, if the 1976 doctors' strike in Los Angeles is any indication. The doctors unwittingly proved their own dispensability when for an entire month they refused to treat any but the most severe emergencies. The resulting change in the death rate must have alarmed many M.D.'s: It dropped from 21 to as low as 14 a week. Some of the drop was probably due to a lack of elective surgery; fewer people faced operating room hazards, so fewer died.

Another surprise: A survey taken afterward found that the strike appeared to have caused "relatively slight inconvenience to the people of Los Angeles."

the Rehabilitation Institute of Chicago teaches people that to feel good, they must help themselves. Many people who have suffered from long-term, "incurable" low back pain have found relief—without drugs, surgery or complicated equipment—by practicing the center's home exercise therapy.

After careful diagnosis, the patients are taught simple whole-body exercises that strengthen the body and reduce pain. They are taught the proper way to lift heavy objects, and to recognize the early signs of trouble before they develop into backaches.

According to Robert G. Addison, M.D., founder of the center, more than 75 percent of those who learn the therapy report significant improvement at home. The trick is to stick with the exercises. The center can only teach patients; it can't exercise for them. The self-reliance patients learn also gives them a needed psychological boost, says Dr. Addison. (Chapter 2 of this book will teach you other ways to protect yourself against backaches.)

Controlling High Blood Pressure

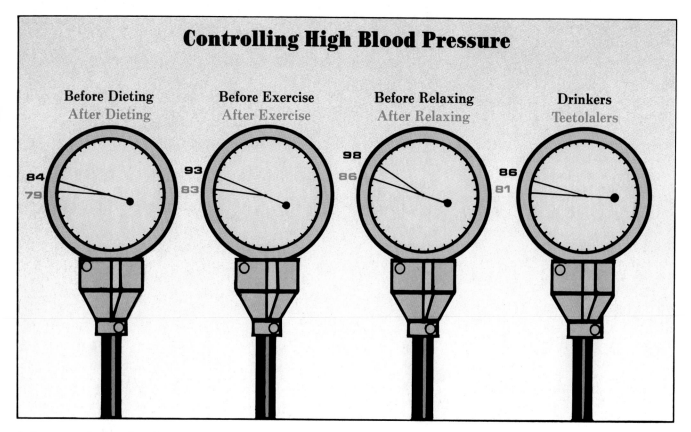

| Before Dieting | Before Exercise | Before Relaxing | Drinkers |
| After Dieting | After Exercise | After Relaxing | Teetolalers |

84
79

93
83

98
86

86
81

A drug prescription almost always follows the diagnosis of high blood pressure. But like many of the conditions discussed in this book, mild high blood pressure can be controlled without drugs—and with self-care. These studies prove the point. (They all measured diastolic blood pressure, the second number in the reading.)

—A University of Minnesota School of Public Health study found that 82 overweight men who dieted for a 10 percent weight loss lowered their blood pressure from means of 84 to 79.

—Hypertensive patients in Mississippi lowered their readings from 93 to 83 after 3 months of aerobic exercise.

—Relaxation training helped 19 Stanford University subjects lower their rate from 98 to 86.

—Researchers in Australia found that a test group of men who didn't drink had a mean diastolic rate of 81, while drinkers were measured at 86.

All these pressure-lowering lifestyle changes can be done by *you*—without expensive equipment, doctors or medications.

STUDENT TEACHERS

Simple self-care education has also proved useful at many schools like the University of Southern California, Los Angeles, where students help each other learn a lesson as important as any their professors will teach: How to safeguard their own health. Amy Zimmerman Dale, M.P.H., director of health education at the USC Student Health and Counseling Service, says that "many students are bewildered by medical problems because it's their first time away from the family. At home, Mom often took care of all the doctor's appointments and health problems. A lot of students don't even know how to take their own temperature when they come to USC."

In response to this problem, Ms. Dale has established a training program where interested students are taught all aspects of first aid and general health maintenance, including nutrition. Students are encouraged to visit these "health advocates" for health advice. If a student has a cold, for example, a health advocate will explain how to treat the symptoms and suggest that the student try warm liquids and lots of rest instead of a visit to a doctor. The health advocates also hand out health pamphlets written especially for college-age people. "Our goal is to educate people so they'll see themselves as partners with their doctors," says Ms. Dale.

CHILDREN NOT IMMUNE FROM BENEFITS

Learning self-care shouldn't be postponed until children start college, however. "Self-care education is very valid in pediatrics," says James E. Strain, M.D., former president of the American Academy of Pediatrics, now in private practice and a clinical professor of pediatrics at the University of Colorado, Denver. "Parents should learn when to call a doctor and when to treat the child at home."

When Junior gets sick, many parents find it easiest to run straight to the pediatrician, but sometimes parents do as good a job as health professionals in managing their children's illness.

According to Robert S. Mendelsohn, M.D., author of *How to Raise a Healthy Child . . . in Spite of Your Doctor,* "At least 95 percent of the ailments that children are prey to will heal themselves and do not require medical attention." He recommends that parents become well informed by reading books and talking to their doctors. That way they'll know when to treat the child themselves and when to see a doctor.

Dr. Strain agrees: "If I can teach a parent to be self-sufficient and comfortable with self-care, then I've fulfilled my goal. This is a very important part of pediatrics."

LEARN TO BREATHE AT CAMP WHEEZ

Asthmatic children at "Camp Wheez," in Palo Alto, California, offer further evidence that pediatrics and self-care go hand in hand. Asthma is a commonly misunderstood disease, and, sadly, a lack of knowledge about it can cause many people much unnecessary trauma. A survey of children at the camp found that most underestimated their lung capacity and knew little about the causes of asthma, including the influence of emotions and the effects of medications. The parents weren't much more knowledgeable: More than half were unaware of the causes of asthma, including the fact that allergens contribute to the problem. Between 6 and 12 months after completing the program, which taught self-help skills, 73 percent of the parents noted that their children were following their treatment program better and had fewer emergency room visits due to their asthma.

AVOIDING DENTAL PAIN

It's easy to cringe at the sound of a dental drill—even when we're still in

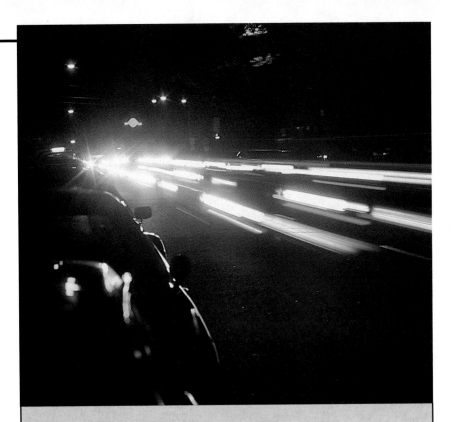

Seat Belts: Self-Care at 55 Miles per Hour

Although few of us think of seat belts as self-care tools, they outperform stethoscopes and speculums in saving lives. Experts polled by Louis Harris on the most important things adults can do to protect their health ranked wearing seat belts 4th. Not driving after drinking was ranked 5th (drunk driving accounts for over 50 percent of all auto fatalities) and driving within the speed limit was 23rd.

Here's why buckling up is such an important part of self-care:
- You are likely to be involved in a crash once every 5 years.
- Three out of four accidents happen within 25 miles of home.
- Slamming into the windshield when your car is moving at 30 miles per hour generates more impact than jumping headfirst off a 2-story building.

If we all chose to use seat belts, 14,000 to 18,000 needless deaths would be prevented each year. There would also be over a million fewer cases of mutilation and paralysis from car accidents.

So cultivate an important health habit. Next time you get behind the wheel, take a moment to buckle up and urge your passengers to follow suit.

the waiting room. We imagine the pain, the helplessness—and the looming face of the dentist, who seems almost eager to jack-hammer away at our molars.

But dental work—and gum surgery in particular—isn't always necessary, according to Clifford M. Wilk, D.D.S., a Chicago dentist who likes to be "partners" with his patients. He has developed a new way for patients to prevent gingivitis, an inflammation of the gums often caused by plaque and bacteria buildup.

Many dentists are quick to strip gums when treating the disease, but Dr. Wilk advocates "dry brushing" to remove the plaque and tartar which contribute to gingivitis. Toothpaste, says Dr. Wilk, is a cosmetic. It's fine for freshening

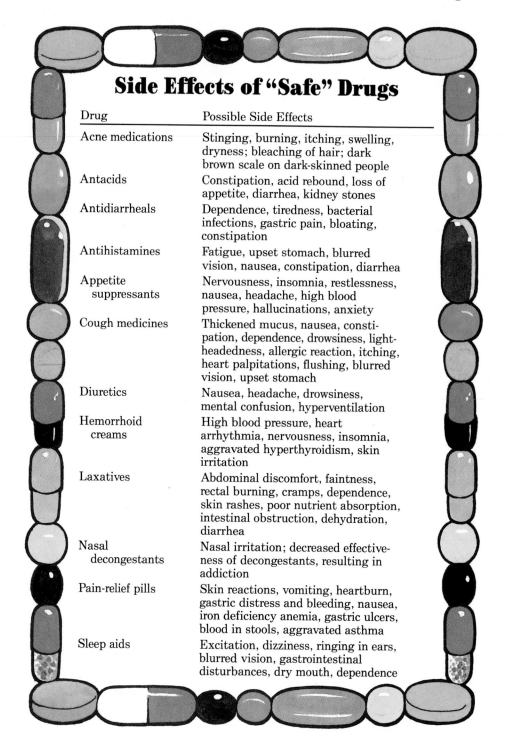

Side Effects of "Safe" Drugs

Drug	Possible Side Effects
Acne medications	Stinging, burning, itching, swelling, dryness; bleaching of hair; dark brown scale on dark-skinned people
Antacids	Constipation, acid rebound, loss of appetite, diarrhea, kidney stones
Antidiarrheals	Dependence, tiredness, bacterial infections, gastric pain, bloating, constipation
Antihistamines	Fatigue, upset stomach, blurred vision, nausea, constipation, diarrhea
Appetite suppressants	Nervousness, insomnia, restlessness, nausea, headache, high blood pressure, hallucinations, anxiety
Cough medicines	Thickened mucus, nausea, constipation, dependence, drowsiness, lightheadedness, allergic reaction, itching, heart palpitations, flushing, blurred vision, upset stomach
Diuretics	Nausea, headache, drowsiness, mental confusion, hyperventilation
Hemorrhoid creams	High blood pressure, heart arrhythmia, nervousness, insomnia, aggravated hyperthyroidism, skin irritation
Laxatives	Abdominal discomfort, faintness, rectal burning, cramps, dependence, skin rashes, poor nutrient absorption, intestinal obstruction, dehydration, diarrhea
Nasal decongestants	Nasal irritation; decreased effectiveness of decongestants, resulting in addiction
Pain-relief pills	Skin reactions, vomiting, heartburn, gastric distress and bleeding, nausea, iron deficiency anemia, gastric ulcers, blood in stools, aggravated asthma
Sleep aids	Excitation, dizziness, ringing in ears, blurred vision, gastrointestinal disturbances, dry mouth, dependence

We often reach for over-the-counter remedies for our minor aches, sniffles or itches without thinking twice. After all, drugstores couldn't stock anything that could harm us. Or could they?

Many familiar products can trigger unwanted side effects, even if you use them according to directions. Here's a list of the most common side effects of ordinary drugstore remedies. You can minimize the likelihood of side effects by reading labels and package inserts carefully before using the product.

your breath and mouth but often gets in the way of removing plaque from the teeth. What you need to do is brush your gums carefully, but rather vigorously, for 5 minutes a day. Use a soft brush with thin bristles that have rounded and polished ends. "Lying in bed is a good place for dry brushing," he says, "because then saliva will collect in the base of the throat instead of wetting your brush." He recommends placing the bristles at a 45-degree angle where the gum meets the tooth, and then moving the brush back and forth ¼ inch at a time. After brushing, says Dr. Wilk, run dental floss around each tooth to remove all the plaque that has accumulated there. Unless plaque is brushed away every 24 hours, it will harden into tartar that could cause gingivitis.

The whole procedure takes about 5 minutes, but the benefits will last a lifetime. And you won't spend money paying unnecessary dental bills.

PUTTING THE HURT ON HICCUPS

Unfortunately, some doctors take their faith in technology to such an extreme that their logic becomes even harder to understand than their handwriting. A case of hiccups, for example, is transformed by many doctors from a problem easily treated at home to a high-tech headache. These doctors treat prolonged hiccups by massaging the back of the roof of the mouth with a rubber suction catheter, a procedure that is "at least mildly unpleasant and would require the availability of such a catheter and a certain degree of medical expertise" (not to mention an expensive office visit), writes Steven Goldsmith, M.D., in the *Journal of the American Medical Association.*

According to Dr. Goldsmith, people can sidestep these problems by learning simple, less intrusive treatments that can be performed at home without the "benefit" of

catheters, doctors and office fees (see chapter 5 for some specific suggestions). And what's true for hiccups is true for most of the health problems covered in this book.

LET'S GET FISCAL

Twenty-four percent of the people surveyed by the American Hospital Association felt that doctors' fees accounted for the rising costs of their care. Tests like X rays are an added expense that can make a visit to the doctor as costly as a weekend in Las Vegas. But Donald Vickery, M.D., president of the Center for Consumer Health Education in Reston, Virginia, says that self-care can reduce visits to the doctor by 17 percent overall. And if only minor illnesses are counted, the reduction can be as much as 35 percent. Clearly, self-care is a good way to beat the rising cost of health care, which could reach $600 billion by 1987 in America alone—well over $2,000 a year per person.

The primary tool people use to learn about health and self-care is the written word, and dollar for dollar, health-care literature saves people money. Dr. Vickery estimates that a self-care book costing $2 has reduced visits to the doctor enough to save each reader an average of $39. That's about a 20-to-1 return on investment.

We hope you'll consider *Every-day Health Hints* an investment in your own self-care. Whether you suffer the aches and pains of everyday life, the miseries of colds and flu, or you simply want to ensure a healthy vacation for yourself and your family, you'll find most of the basic, up-to-date information you'll need right here. You can become self-sufficient in caring for the minor ills and a better partner for your doctor should a major one arise. We'll tell you when and how to treat yourself at home and when it's time to seek professional help. Once you're armed with the information in this book, you'll be well on your way to becoming independently healthy for life.

Self-Care Tools

Numerous tools are now available to make self-care easier and more comprehensive than in the past. New devices are coming out at a rapid clip—many equal in accuracy and quality to those used in hospitals. Peruse the items listed here for initial health-care ideas. (See the Buyer's Guide on page 162 for catalog and ordering information.)

Children's Stethoscope

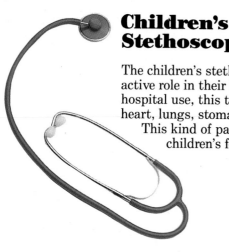

The children's stethoscope lets young people take an active role in their health care. Accurate enough for hospital use, this tool allows kids to listen to the heart, lungs, stomach—every part of the body. This kind of participation helps lessen children's fear of doctors and nurses.

Otoscope with Dental Mirror

Parents can check for ear infections in their children with this safe, simple and reliable otoscope. Problems can be discovered and treated before they become serious. The penlight handle and mirror also can be used for dental self-exams.

Vitamin C Self-Test Kit

With this kit you can accurately test your body's vitamin C levels in just a few minutes. You can see how stress affects vitamin C in the body and determine how much of the vitamin you need to keep your cells and immune system in top shape.

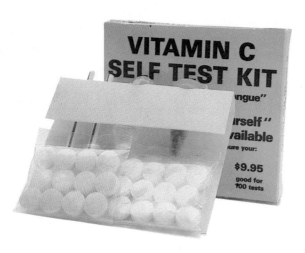

VITAMIN C
SELF TEST KIT

"...ngue"

...rself"

...vailable

...ure your:

$9.95

good for
700 tests

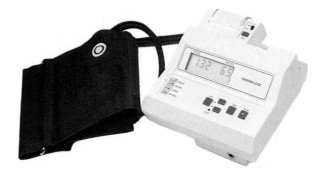

Norelco Blood Pressure Kit

Studies have shown that home blood pressure testing is more accurate than that done at the doctor's office. This digital blood pressure monitor enables everyone to find out if they are among the approximately 1 in 5 Americans who suffer from high blood pressure. And it's great for monitoring the effects of blood pressure treatments, too.

Microstix-Nitrite Test

Save yourself time, money and discomfort with these easy-to-use strips that aid in the detection of cystitis or other urinary tract infections. The home test gives your doctor the option of prescribing the proper treatment over the phone.

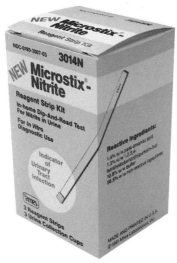

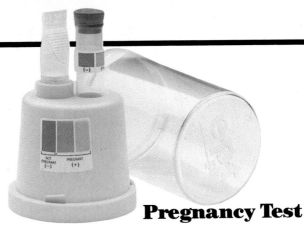

Pregnancy Test

Home pregnancy tests offer privacy and convenience by allowing you to check for the hormone excreted by the developing placenta. Positive results are 98 percent accurate and mean a baby is probably on the way. A negative result is slightly less accurate, so you may want to repeat the test for reassurance.

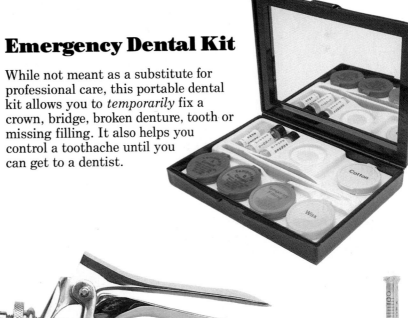

Emergency Dental Kit

While not meant as a substitute for professional care, this portable dental kit allows you to *temporarily* fix a crown, bridge, broken denture, tooth or missing filling. It also helps you control a toothache until you can get to a dentist.

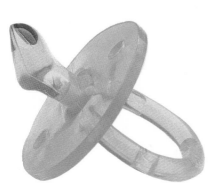

Baby Temperature Thermometer

This pacifier can be doubly comforting to a baby and its parents because it constantly and safely monitors body temperature while eliminating the need for a rectal thermometer, as well as performing the normal function of a pacifier. The temperature dot changes from green to black when the baby's temperature rises above 100°. The pacifier is nontoxic, safe and easily sterilized.

Vaginal Speculum and Basal Body Thermometer

Vaginal self-exams help women understand their anatomy, identify various infections and determine which days of the menstrual cycle are fertile. The speculum makes a vaginal self-exam simple. The basal body thermometer registers temperature changes associated with ovulation, to make it easier to determine fertile times. Both tools give women greater control of their gynecological health.

2

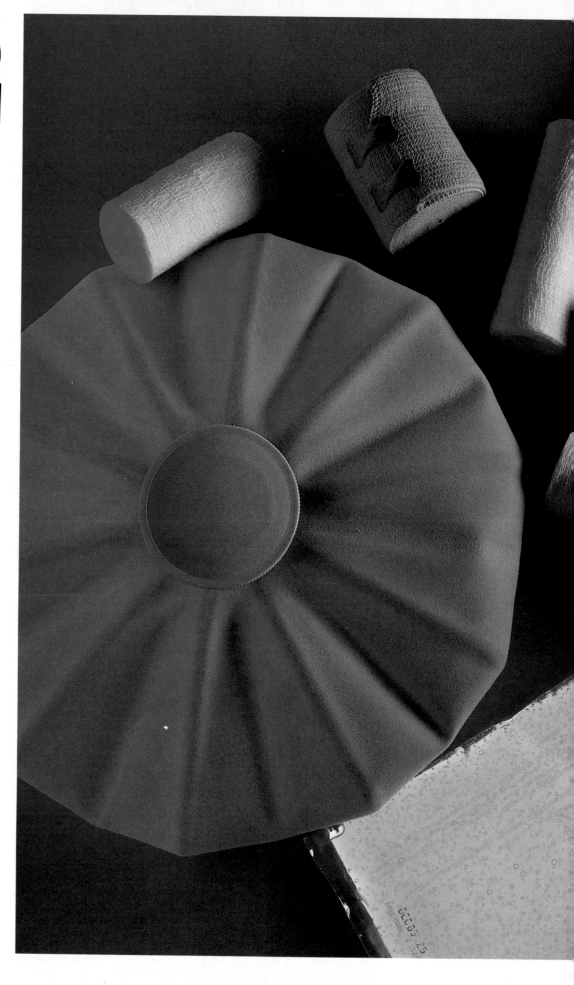

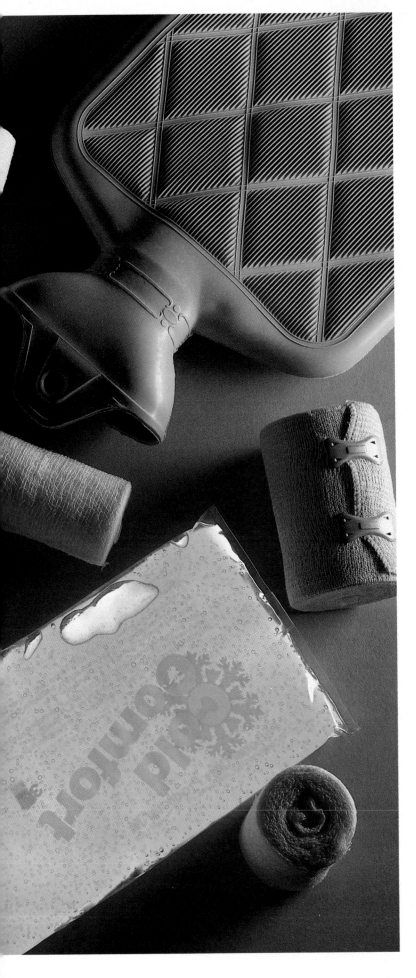

Easing Aches and Pains

You can draw on your body's own natural resources to relieve the aches and pains of everyday life.

E d and Cheryl were on their way to a party. Halfway there—15 miles from home—Ed swore out loud. Next thing Cheryl knew, the car screeched into a U-turn. She didn't even ask Ed why he'd turned back—she knew he was going to get his Fiorinal, a potent headache medication. Cheryl worries about her husband but she knows how she feels with painful menstrual cramps.

Like Ed and Cheryl, millions of Americans suffer from pain. "Oh, my aching back" is practically a national anthem. And in that same repertoire are headaches, sore feet, muscle and menstrual cramps.

But pain itself isn't the enemy. In fact, it's a kind of friend, telling us that something's wrong. That means that while an occasional aspirin can help, dosing with drugs can also mask the cause of pain—and yet only when you know the cause can you do something about it.

Researchers agree that pain is a neural signal that enters the spinal column at points called nerve gates. Analgesic drugs can close off nerve gates, easing pain. But scientists have further discovered that the human body houses its own pharmacy of natural opiates, called endorphins, that serve the same purpose. A shiatsu massage for a migraine, for example, is thought to set off endorphin release. Massage, warm baths, ice packs, acupressure and a daily jog are all capable of stimulating the body to release its own natural painkillers.

This means that using a wide array of nondrug therapies—like the kind you'll read about in this chapter—can do much to help free the body from common aches and pains.

Headaches

Of every three patients visiting a doctor, one complains of headaches, and fully 90 percent of all Americans get headaches at some point. That's a lot of discomfort. At least modern doctors don't use a remedy popular among medieval physicians, who drilled holes in their patients' skulls to let the headache-causing demons out. In fact, today's most up-to-date headache treatments stress headache management—learning how to *avoid* headaches in the first place. And that means knowing *why* you get them. Seymour Diamond, M.D., of the Diamond Headache Clinic in Chicago, recommends that sufferers of chronic headaches keep a log. Whenever a headache hits, you record when it began, how long it lasts, which area of the head is painful and the circumstances surrounding it—stress, diet, menstrual cycle, even the weather. The log will help you and your doctor see if the headaches follow a pattern.

Nine times out of ten, according to Dr. Diamond, the major headache trigger is emotional tension.

Brush Your Headache Away

Want to give your headache the brush-off? The only equipment you'll need is a good hairbrush or bath brush with fairly stiff natural bristles, says biophysicist Harry C. Ehrmantraut, Ph.D., inventor of "brush therapy" for headaches. Starting at the temples, just above the eyebrows, rotate the brush in small circles about ½ inch in diameter, moving up-back-down-and-forward (the upper part of the circle should go toward the back of your head). Brushing along the lines shown here, continue pressing the bristles against the skin in little circles. Focus

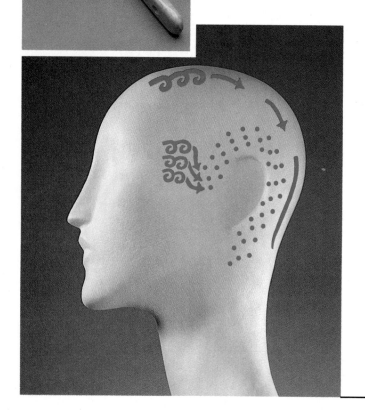

especially on the base of the skull. Also, says Dr. Ehrmantraut, "be sure to pay attention with careful brushing to the uppermost point in front of the ear. The main artery supplying the scalp runs through this area, where it also intersects the main chewing muscles of the jaw. Since we often clench our jaw when we're tense, the resulting congestion becomes most painful here."

How does the technique work? The rotating strokes stimulate the tissues lying beneath the skin's surface, says Dr. Ehrmantraut, allowing for better blood circulation and, consequently, a better supply of oxygen.

THE TENSION HEADACHE: PAIN IN A TIGHT SPOT

When you're tense—anxious or frustrated, or holding your body in one position too long—the muscles in your head and neck knot up. That irritates the sensitive nerve endings in tissues surrounding the blood vessels, causing pain. Headache experts agree that practically *anything* you can do to relieve stress will help ease tension headaches.

Getting regular exercise scores high in easing stress. Relaxation training and biofeedback can also help many people stay headache free, says Stewart Agras, Ph.D., a Stanford University psychiatrist. "And for some," he adds, "just taking a warm bath is a good substitute for aspirin."

And Dr. Diamond believes that sometimes people just "need to learn how to say no" so they don't take on more responsibilities, projects—and stress—than they can handle.

Even so, there are times when heavy-duty stress is unavoidable—when *not* getting a headache would seem nothing short of a miracle.

Kazuyuki Matsuo, Ph.D., knows what that's all about. One of the top simultaneous interpreters in the world, Dr. Matsuo has often been an English "voice" for high-ranking Japanese officials. On a stress scale of 1 to 10, his job rates a 9½. By the time he gets home after an assignment, he's ripe for a whopper of a headache.

His wife, Linda, goes to work massaging his feet the minute he steps out of his shoes. "In a half hour, he is completely relaxed," she says. "I never give the headache a chance, if I can help it."

The feet do indeed have a hotline to the head, says Laura Norman, a foot reflexologist from New York City who massages feet for a living. She explains that various reflex areas on the foot correspond to points on the whole body so that "just by massaging the feet, you can totally relax the whole body." For tension headaches, she says, "Concentrate on the toes—

especially the big toe—and the base of the toes. Press with the outer edge of the thumb, bending the joint and inching along the foot." Similarly, Japanese acupressure focuses on trigger points (see "Press Here for Headache Relief" on page 15).

To loosen stiff shoulders, which aggravate tension headaches, apply a hot pack made by soaking a towel in hot water and wringing it out. Having someone massage your sore shoulders and upper back also breaks up tension.

THE MIGRAINE HEADACHE: SKULL-DUGGERY

"How does a migraine feel? I'd rather tell you how it feels when it's *gone,* when I can get out of bed and walk around without stumbling into a bureau or door, when I can open my curtains and welcome the sunlight in again, when my son calling 'Mommy' sounds like sweet music to my ears. At first, I can never quite believe it's finally over. It's funny, but I always go look in the mirror—maybe to make sure that half my head hasn't exploded away. I'm just totally wiped out after the headache's gone. I feel sort of like a war veteran: battle-weary, yet thrilled to make it back alive."

Only a migraine sufferer can describe a migraine. Those were the words of a woman who has had migraines since age 17. She's not alone, by any means.

Nearly 10 percent of all Americans suffer migraines, headaches that are classed as vascular—that is, having to do with the blood vessels. In the migraine—for reasons as yet unexplained—blood vessels in the head first constrict, then dilate sharply, pressing against neighboring nerve endings. In practically no time flat, an excruciatingly painful, throbbing headache takes over half the head, often centering behind one eye. (The word "migraine" comes from the Greek *hemi,* or "half," and *crania,* which means "head.") Sometimes a migraine will attack first one side of the head and then seem to move to the other side. In some cases, a migraine will blitz both sides at once for a double whammy. The attack can last for hours or even days.

There are two types of migraine: classic and common. People who have classic migraine know when a headache is brewing because the pain is preceded by an aura, or set of warning signals. They may see flashing lights or blind spots in their field of vision, suffer mild confusion and become abnormally sensitive to otherwise moderate levels of sound and light. In common migraine (which afflicts 80 percent of migraine sufferers), there is no aura, although some people report feeling irritable and depressed before the migraine sets in.

A migraine is sometimes called a sick headache, since nausea and vomiting may accompany the torturous pain. It's enough to send a person to bed—and that's exactly where most migraine sufferers end up, trying to sleep it off. Like a wounded animal, migraine sufferers head for the solitude of their own private "cave" (usually the bedroom) where all light and sound can be blocked out, with a bag or two of ice to place on the thumping temples.

There's wisdom in that instinct, it seems. Headache experts concur that migraine-prone people tend to drive themselves too hard and may well need plenty of rest. But they also agree that such forced retirement isn't the best way to cope. Far better, they say, to help prevent migraines by including plenty of rest and plenty of stress relievers in your life. The advice of most headache clinics: Get regular exercise, practice some form of relaxation or meditation, and even schedule in one day a week when you have nothing to do but take it easy.

If migraines persist, the next step often recommended is biofeedback training, one of the most remarkable nondrug techniques for treating and preventing migraines. Biofeedback uses electronic equipment to teach people how they can control blood flow simply by mental

concentration. Its use for migraine was discovered accidentally at the Menninger Clinic, when a woman with a severe migraine was suddenly freed from pain at exactly the same moment she mentally directed a great deal of blood flow to her hands. Further research has shown that such "hand-warming" techniques work well, by diverting blood flow away from the swollen arteries in the head.

Using biofeedback and cutting back on stress are good ways to cut back on migraines. But even these may fail to keep migraines at bay if you are one of the many people who suffer from migraines triggered by food.

THE ANTIMIGRAINE DIET

"At least 25 to 30 percent of migraine sufferers are helped by dietary strategy," says Dr. Diamond.

Foods like chocolate, aged cheese and red wine are notorious for triggering migraines in sensitive individuals. All contain substances called amines, which can cause blood vessels to swell. Peanuts, salt, fresh yeasted breads, citrus fruits, meats and cheeses cured with nitrites, alcohol, pork, lima beans and navy beans are also known to bring on migraines.

Joan Miller, Ph.D., a headache specialist from Atlanta, Georgia, says that the best way to find out if you're food sensitive is to experiment by cutting out foods that you suspect, one at a time. The problem is that you must be patient and persistent. Some headaches show up as much as a day or two after an offending food is eaten. And sometimes a combination of foods may trigger a headache.

On top of that, stress may exacerbate food sensitivity. According to Dr. Miller, "Many times you can get away with eating a certain food until you're under some stress, then the food plus the stress equals a migraine. I've had clients who've triggered a headache with a handful of peanuts eaten during a stressful time. Yet two weeks before that they

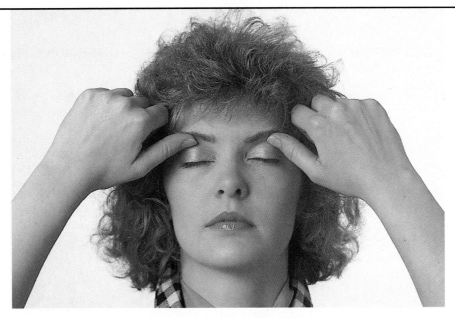

Press Here for Headache Relief

The room is quiet; all you hear is your own deep breathing. Your eyes are closed. You bend your thumbs at right angles, lift them, train them on "trigger points" on your head, and take aim. Then you press in, probing for the sensitive areas that tell you you're on target. Ooo—that hurts. You hold for 15 to 30 seconds, then release. You press again. And again if necessary. Ooo—ouch. Release. Ah. Your head feels much better now. Ah, so. Japanese acupressure (shiatsu) proves itself once more.

Acupressure is a cousin to acupuncture, the Oriental medical art that says lines of energy, or meridians, connect the various parts of the body like subway lines, and that by stimulating one point on the line you can relieve a problem or ache anywhere along its track. But where acupuncture stimulates the meridians with tiny needles, acupressure uses finger-pressure massage. You may be able to relieve a sinus headache, for instance, by massaging and pressing the points under the eyebrows (pictured above) that are on a line running through the sinus area. (Western science doesn't accept the existence of meridians, but studies indicate that acupressure stimulates the release of natural painkillers, like endorphins and norepinephrine.)

Instead of the thumb, you can press with your fingers, using the meaty portion of the fingertips. Move in steady circles in and around the points. Better yet, if you have the opportunity, enlist someone to work on the points for you.

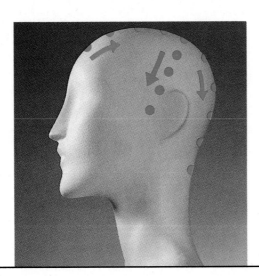

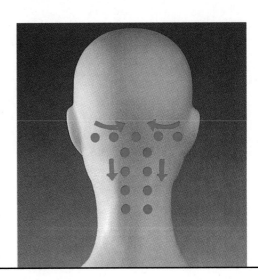

had eaten nuts and *didn't* get a headache."

Although avoiding certain foods can be a useful strategy against migraines, don't avoid food to the point where you skip meals. John Brainard, M.D., whose own migraines prompted him to write a book, *Control of Migraines,* says that low blood sugar— a result of not eating regularly—can also lead to migraine.

As you've probably guessed by now, there are no overnight solutions to managing migraines. But as your awareness of your body's sensitivities increases, you will find the health gains well worth some persistent detective work.

Some migraine triggers are hard to fight: changes in weather or altitude, smoky rooms, pollen, mold and perfume, to name a few. Also,

fluctuating estrogen levels can bring on a headache, which explains why many women get migraines during ovulation and menstruation.

In general, more women suffer migraines than men. But men are particularly prone to another type of debilitating vascular headache, the cluster headache.

THE CLUSTER HEADACHE: A BUNCH OF TROUBLE

The searing, stabbing pain of a cluster headache often strikes at night about 90 minutes after retiring or in the wee hours of the morning. The pain tends to center on one eye, which may water and look bloodshot. One nostril may be stuffed or runny, too.

Typically, the headache lasts up to 2 hours and then hits again once, twice or three times in the same day— only to recur the next day as well. The attacks may last from three to eight weeks. Then they disappear altogether, and months may pass before they occur again— hence the name "cluster."

It's hard to treat a cluster headache once it's begun, but there have been several encouraging reports of relief obtained with a rather unorthodox therapy: vigorous exercise. Cluster victims will find that it's far more constructive to do jumping jacks or run in place than to try tearing doors off their hinges while in the clutches of a cluster. (Doctors report that desperate patients not only wrestle with doors but plead with people nearby to knock them out—the pain is that intense.) For some reason, exercise that raises the heart rate can ease cluster headache pain, possibly due to endorphins released during vigorous activity, or increased oxygen flow to the blood vessels. (Interestingly, though, such exercise during a migraine attack will only make the migraine worse.)

But if you're in a cluster period (when clusters strike daily), be careful not to run or engage in strenuous exercise *between* attacks, says Lee Kudrow, M.D., director of

Shower Your Headache Away

Head your headache for the showers—first a hot one, then a cold one—and stay in until you shiver, says Augustus S. Rose, M.D. This professor emeritus at the UCLA School of Medicine found that many of his patients' migraines could be washed right down the drain this way. You may find you need to repeat the alternating showers, but at the very least, the pain may lessen considerably. Here's why: Hot water causes the blood vessels to dilate widely (which may initially intensify the migraine). The cold water then shocks the blood vessels into constricting, so they exert less pressure on adjacent nerves. After all, the cause of pain in migraine is that very pressure. Dr. Rose adds that if you're lucky enough to be near a cold pool or the ocean, a quick plunge at the first twinges of pain works just as well as showering. For anyone who has experienced the hot throb-throb-throbbing of a migraine, Dr. Rose's therapies may be a cold splash of relief.

the California Medical Clinic for Headache. It may then precipitate an attack.

Some cluster patients also benefit from inhaling oxygen from an oxygen tank during an attack—under a doctor's supervision, of course.

In one study, Dr. Kudrow asked 50 cluster patients to compare oxygen therapy with a commonly prescribed drug for cluster, ergotamine tartrate. If the headache pain was stopped or greatly reduced within 15 minutes in seven out of ten attacks, the therapy was deemed successful. Using that standard, oxygen therapy worked for 41 patients, and ergotamine helped 35, giving oxygen the edge as a treatment of choice. Some patients keep tanks both at home and in the office.

To date, there are no sure cures for cluster headaches. But in searching for ways to prevent them, research has uncovered two big don'ts: Don't smoke and don't drink alcohol. Both habits are closely linked to this ailment.

THE SINUS HEADACHE: UNDRAINED PAIN

Practically everyone who's ever had a head cold has experienced a sinus headache. The nose feels full, there is a slicing pain in the cheekbones, the bridge of the nose is swollen and sore, the head aches with a dull, unrelenting throb. It's an absolutely miserable sensation.

Fortunately, sinus headaches that recur, or attack chronically, are rare, according to headache experts. In fact, says Dr. Diamond, migraines and clusters are often misdiagnosed as sinus headaches. In true sinus headache, the mucous linings of the sinus cavities are engorged and inflamed. Mucus can't drain properly since the sinus ducts are blocked. You may be feverish, and your teeth may hurt, too. Typically, the headache pain begins its assault

in the morning—after fluids have backed up in the sinuses overnight—and grows more severe as the day wears on. At night, it lets up. Unlike migraine, lying down only makes a sinus headache worse.

There's not much you can do to prevent sinus headaches. They're caused by infections, nasal polyps, or anatomical problems that obstruct the sinus ducts (such as a deviated septum). For some people, they kick up during hay fever season.

As you've probably guessed by now, sinus headaches are the type of ailment that requires a doctor. Treatment ranges from antibiotics, decongestants and antihistamines to surgical drainage, in severe cases. There are some simple, nondrug measures you can take, however, that reduce the pain and also promote drainage and help you get through the day comfortably.

The best remedy is lounging in a steam bath, but if you can't get to one, try a warm pack draped across the eyes and cheekbones. To prepare one, take a thick, fluffy washcloth, soak it in very warm (not hot) water, wring it out and drape it on the painful area. As soon as it cools off, warm it up again and reapply. Keep this up for about 10 minutes or until you feel relief. Many people say it's best to sit down for this therapy and tip your head forward somewhat to let the sinuses drain through the nose, so that you don't have uncomfortable post-nasal drip in the back of the throat as the mucus loosens up.

Another helpful technique is to use a steam vaporizer or run a hot shower and sit in the steamy bathroom.

For the best results of all, combine one or more of these methods with finger-pressure massage (see "Press Here for Headache Relief" on page 15). It's worth a try—especially since you may be taking a decongestant or other drug for the sinus condition, and you may feel reluctant to take a painkiller on top of that.

Run Away from Headaches

Have you ever tried to run away from your headaches?

Headache specialist Seymour Diamond, M.D., says that running could help alleviate the symptoms of several different kinds of headaches.

"For people who find running relaxing, it could relieve a muscle tension headache," he says. "And vigorous exercise sometimes brings relief of a cluster headache, so I recommend running during an attack.

"Finally, there's a theory that running increases the production of endorphins, the body's natural painkillers," Dr. Diamond adds, "so a regular running program could lessen the pain of a migraine headache."

Dr. Diamond stresses that a running program should be implemented gradually because each individual will react differently.

Exercises for Headache Relief

Doctors and dentists have found that head, neck and shoulder muscles can be thrown out of alignment due to postural and jaw problems. The result: headaches. Lawrence A. Funt, D.D.S., M.S.D., of the Cranio-Facial Pain Center in Bethesda, Maryland, developed the following easy stretches to help relieve tension in the neck, shoulders and back, and prevent these headaches.

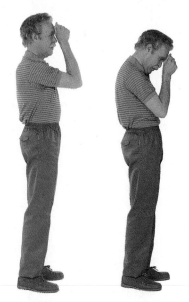

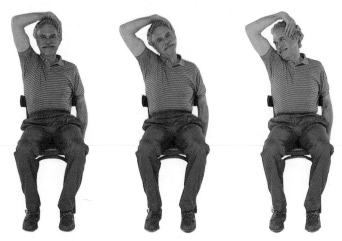

Tilt and Turn

This exercise stretches the front muscles of your chest and neck. Sit straight in a chair, supporting the left side of your body by gripping the edge of your chair with your left arm. Raise your right hand and gently rest it on your left temple. Tilt your head toward your right shoulder until the muscles on the left side of your neck start to pull. Stop, and slowly turn your head so that your nose points toward the right elbow and you feel muscles start to tug. Continue tilting your head toward your right shoulder as far as is comfortable. Repeat on the left side. Do this sequence 3 times a day.

Sky Watch

This also stretches the front of the neck and chest. Sit straight, but relaxed, in a chair. Lean your head back as though you were looking at the sky and slowly open your mouth wide. Let your upper body move; don't put all the pressure on your neck. Do this exercise 3 times a day.

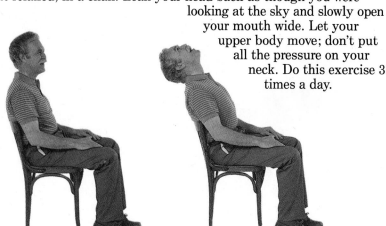

Forehead Support

This exercise will stretch your back and neck muscles. Make a fist with one hand and place it thumbside-in against your forehead, so it supports your head completely. Drop your head forward very slowly until you feel the muscles start to pull. Then stop. Be sure your fist is giving adequate support. Do this exercise 3 times a day.

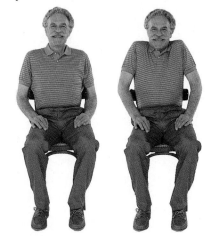

Shrug

Sit straight in a chair with your hands on your lap. Raise your shoulders toward your ears as far as is comfortable and hold for 2 seconds. Drop your shoulders 1 inch and hold for 2 more seconds. Then drop your shoulders back to the normal position. This relaxes all your upper-body muscles. Do this exercise 3 times a day.

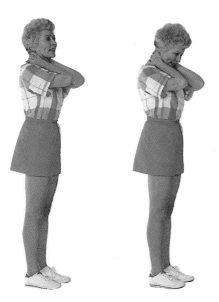
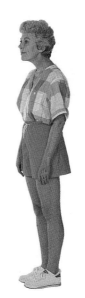
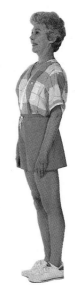

Short Yes Stretch

This stretch will loosen your upper neck muscles and ligaments and make you feel less stiff. First, place both hands behind your neck with fingers entwined. Move your head forward slowly and gently 6 times as if you're nodding yes.

Turkey Peck

The turkey peck works on your lower neck by loosening the joints. Start with your head upright and your chin jutting out straight ahead from your neck. Then slowly move your head until your chin is pulled in like a soldier's. Breathe in deeply through your nose only. Do this exercise 6 times.

Thumbs-Out Shoulder Roll

To stretch your chest muscles, roll your shoulders forward gently, keeping your arms loosely at your sides. As you roll your shoulders up and back, rotate your hands 180 degrees, keeping your thumbs pointed out from your palms.

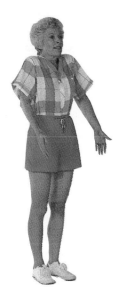
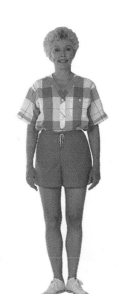
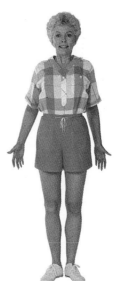
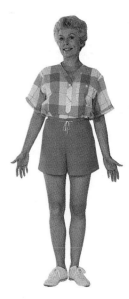

Putting It All Together

This gives you the full effect of the turkey peck and the shoulder roll. Stand up straight with your heels together. Slowly and gently, do the thumbs-out shoulder roll, and finish with the turkey peck. Repeat the sequence 6 times.

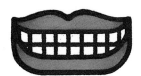

20 Unsuspected Causes of Headache

1 The Gnasher Headache

Nocturnal grinding and clenching of teeth can leave you feeling as though your head is in a vise. Four out of five gnashers are women, and some find that calcium supplements and relaxation techniques solve the problem.

2 The Cocktail Headache

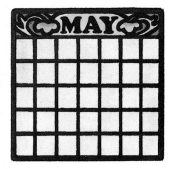

Sometimes it takes only a few drinks to cause a major headache. It depends on how sensitive you are to toxins that collect in the body after a night on the town. Aspirin may irritate a stomach already inflamed by alcohol, so try a cold shower to constrict the swollen, aching blood vessels in your head.

MAY

4 The Caffeine Headache

When your usual daily dose of coffee, soda or other caffeine source is withheld, blood vessels in the head dilate and pain ensues. Cut back gradually on caffeine to avoid this problem.

5 The Hot Dog Headache

Food additives called nitrates and nitrites found in hot dogs, cured meats and luncheon meats cause this headache. Read the labels and buy meats that are free of these chemicals.

3 The Premenstrual Headache

Just what you need: a headache along with your cramps and discomfort. These recurring headaches are probably due to water retention by the brain tissues. Some women find relief after taking vitamin B_6.

6 The Ice Cream Headache

Cold foods can overstimulate the nerves in the roof of the mouth, causing headache. Eat or sip slowly and you won't suffer.

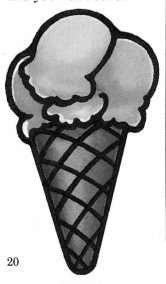

7 The Salt Headache

Migraines sometimes occur several hours after a person eats a salty meal. Try withholding salt from your diet to see if you are susceptible. If you are, season with herbs as you gradually cut back on your salt intake. Enjoy the fresh taste of unsalted food.

8 The Hunger Headache

Avoid this type of between-meal headache, which is caused by low blood sugar, by eating frequent, smaller meals and snacks. Choose high-protein foods like peanuts, yogurt or sunflower seeds. Fresh fruits are also good.

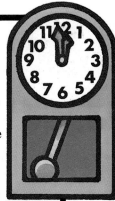

9 The Turtle Headache

When you pull your head under the covers to sleep like a turtle, you don't get enough oxygen. The result: a headache. The cure: fresh air, above the blanket.

10 The Sun Headache

Too much sun can deplete the fluids around the brain and spinal column, causing a headache. Avoid the 11 A.M. to 2 P.M. sun, or wear a hat. If you still get a headache, replace the lost fluids slowly with warm drinks.

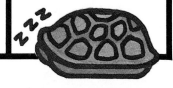

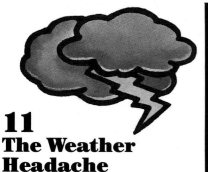

11 The Weather Headache

Changes in the weather may cause a storm in your head. A Swedish study found that certain people tend to suffer headaches just prior to windy weather. Of course, you can't change Mother Nature, but you can limit other factors, like stress and alcohol.

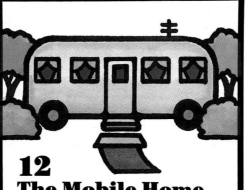

12 The Mobile Home Headache

Mobile homes are often built with materials that release high levels of formaldehyde into the air, causing headaches. Some new regular houses have the same problem. The best remedy: Move, and buy a home that is over 4 years old, the amount of time it takes for the formaldehyde to dissipate.

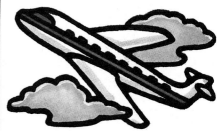

13 The Jet-Set Headache

High levels of ozone in high-flying jets have been shown to cause headaches in passengers. The antioxidants vitamins E and C and selenium and bioflavonoids may help relieve altitude problems.

14 The Snow Shoveler's Headache

These result from blood vessels that don't expand fast enough to handle the stepped-up blood flow that occurs when you do uncustomary exercise, like shoveling snow. Try warming up slowly, especially if you are an erratic exerciser.

15 The Slumber Party Headache

Caused by staying up late and sleeping late when you aren't used to such behavior. The cure: an inviting mattress.

16 The Spike Heel Headache

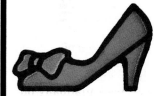

This fashionable headache happens when high heels force the back muscles to tense to keep the body erect. Low heels will solve the problem.

17 The Expressway Headache

This type is similar to turtle headache, but the carbon monoxide comes from rush-hour traffic. Try to adjust your schedule to avoid the pack.

18 The Art Gallery Headache

Not caused by bad art but by simple fatigue brought on by a day spent touring every gallery and museum in town. Minimalist approach recommended for future outings.

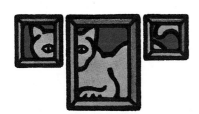

19 The Chinese Food Headache

Symptoms: Throbbing and pressure over the temples and in a band across the forehead. Cause: Monosodium glutamate (MSG), a "flavor enhancer" frequently used in Chinese restaurants. Solution: Tell the waiter to tell the chef to leave out the MSG.

20 The Hat and Goggle Headache

Too much pressure on your forehead and eye sockets can be a real pain. Make sure your swimming goggles are padded; on dry land, don't try to reshape your head with a tight-fitting cap, even if it's the fashionable item this season.

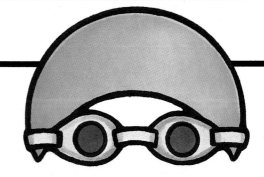

Earaches and Toothaches

Happy Landings— For You and Your Ears

Taking off in a plane doesn't usually cause too many problems. But the landing! That's when air pressure from the cabin is so strong that it creates a vacuum in the middle ear, flattening the eustachian tube. The pain can be overwhelming, unless you do something to restore air pressure in the middle ear. Chewing gum simply doesn't do the trick for some people—but the modified Valsalva's maneuver probably will. Here's how it works: Close your mouth and pinch your nose shut. Then, gently but firmly, blow out your cheeks. If you hear a clicking noise, that's the sound of a successful maneuver. And if at first you don't succeed, give it another try.

"You'd be surprised at what people do to treat pain in their ears," says Frederick Henderson, M.D., of the University of North Carolina in Chapel Hill. "There are all sorts of home remedies. One that's pretty well-known here in the South is warm honey dripped into the ear. But such remedies are not as harmless as people think. In fact, they may well hurt your ear more in the end and obscure the cause of the problem."

A doctor who agrees with this view is Geno J. Merli, M.D., of Jefferson Medical College in Philadelphia. "No home remedy is appropriate for earache," he says. "You should see a doctor for persistent pain."

And that means today, not next week. Left untreated, an infection can lead to hearing loss. But what if you can't see a doctor right away? Is there anything you can do to relieve the pain until your appointment?

Some doctors recommend aspirin or acetaminophen as by far the most useful ways to relieve ear pain, but there are also some nondrug measures you can take. Lying down and elevating the head on a pillow and holding something warm against the ear may make you more comfortable.

LANDING ON YOUR EAR

On an airplane flight, the air on either side of your eardrums—like two passengers sitting next to each other in the cramped coach seats of a typical jet—can't get comfortable. The reason is air pressure. When the plane slides down out of the sky, the air in the middle ear, which normally has plenty of room, is squeezed by the expanding air outside the ear. (At takeoff, it's the inside air that gets rude.) The pushiness jabs the eardrums— and you've got an earache.

How do you get those two to behave—or, in more scientific terms, how do you "equalize the pressure"? One way to prevent airplane earache, or at least minimize discomfort, is to use Valsalva's maneuver (see "Happy Landings— For You and Your Ears"). Don't try it if you have any heart problems, though. Or simply try swallowing, chewing gum or drinking something during the takeoff and landing. These methods help equalize pressure in the inner ear.

If you do order a drink on board, though, make it something other than wine. Audiologist Maurice H. Miller, Ph.D., of New York University and Lenox Hill Hospital, says that histamines in wine can swell tissues in the eustachian tube and upper respiratory tract, making it hard to "pop" the tube and restore normal pressure in the ear. Actually, anything that swells tissues in your head or sinuses, like a sinus infection, a simple cold or an allergy, should make you think twice about flying. If you must fly, consult a physician about taking antihistamines before the trip to reduce the chance of aggravating your ear problems.

TENDING A TOOTHACHE

A persistent, stabbing toothache is almost always caused by decay, which leads to infection in the tooth's pulp. If infection spreads to the tooth's nerve and blood supply, it can cause irreversible damage; the tooth may even die. Left untreated, a dead tooth will eventually abscess and cause still more pain. Obviously, a toothache is nature's pain alarm to wake you up to the fact that it's time to see the dentist. But if the dentist can't see you right away, is there any way to shut off the alarm in the meantime?

"One of the first things people do for pain is to place hot or cold packs on the face, next to the toothache," says Kem Moser, D.D.S., of Kennett Square, Pennsylvania. "If the tooth is dead, hot, moist towels will help. But if it only makes the pain worse, switch to ice packs. If the tooth is alive and infected, and the nerve is inflamed, then cold packs will feel soothing."

If the tooth is still throbbing and you still can't get to a dentist, there's another remedy you might try—clove oil. Ever wonder what dentists use for temporary fillings? They're fillings made of zinc oxide and oil of clove, or eugenol. "Clove oil has an anesthetizing effect on the nerve," says Dr. Moser. "It's something people can use themselves, too, since it's sold over the counter."

Louis P. Gangarosa, D.D.S., Ph.D., of the Medical College of Georgia in Augusta, headed the panel of experts that investigated clove oil for the U.S. Food and Drug Administration, finding it "safe and effective for home use." All you have to do is apply it with a piece of cotton; never introduce the clove oil directly into the mouth using the bottle as a dispenser. One woman who poured clove oil directly on her tooth lost all feeling there— permanently—according to a report in the medical journal *Lancet*.

Another remedy you can try is rinsing your mouth with a warm saline solution (salt and water).

Dr. Moser says that many people place an aspirin directly on an abscessed tooth. But he and other dentists discourage that practice because it can result in "aspirin burns"—raw, painful mouth lesions.

A SENSITIVE SUBJECT

An abscess isn't always at the root of a toothache, so to speak. Sometimes a sinus infection or tense, sore jaw muscles (from clenching the teeth, for example) can mimic toothache. More common, though, is a condition dentists call sensitive teeth: anything from mild to searing pain that occurs whenever something cold, hot, sweet or sour hits the teeth.

"The usual cause of sensitive teeth is overaggressive brushing at the gum line," says Dr. Moser. "As the gum tissue recedes, the roots of teeth are exposed more and more, making the teeth exquisitely and painfully sensitive to certain stimuli."

To avoid this problem, Dr. Moser recommends using a soft-bristled toothbrush, since it cleans better and is unlikely to wear away the gum as medium- or hard-bristled brushes do. He also tells patients to use commercial toothpastes specially made for sensitive teeth. "They have an 85 percent effectiveness rate," he says, "but you have to use them for two

Got a Toothache? Cool It

Take an age-old Chinese therapy for dental pain. Add an ice cube from Western-style physical therapy. Massage well (but gently). What do you get? The best that East and West can offer: a big letup in your toothache, say researchers at McGill University and Montreal General Hospital. They reasoned that ice massage might relieve toothache if concentrated on the *Hoku* point, the trigger point in the web between the thumb and index finger that is needled in Chinese acupuncture to relieve tooth pain. Testing the idea on dental patients in a waiting room— all with acute dental pain— the researchers found that ice massage worked far better to numb pain than *Hoku*-point massage without ice. They theorize that ice massage works by sending super-fast analgesic messages to the brain, which arrive even before messages of tooth pain can register.

weeks before you can feel the benefits. At least one that I know of contains a strontium ion, which binds with molecules on the exposed root surface and provides a kind of 'stucco' coating that desensitizes the tooth."

Dr. Moser also says that diets rich in sugar cause highly acidic saliva that can make teeth sensitive. "Bacteria in plaque metabolize sugar, then secrete acid as a by-product," he explains. Eating too much dried fruit can also cause problems because it's so sticky and sugary, adds Dr. Moser. "Floss *before* as well as after you eat sweet foods. You'll lower the chance that plaque bacteria will interact with sugar." Our suggestion: Avoid sugary foods, saving desserts for special times.

Foot Problems

There are hard hats. And safety goggles with plastic as tough as steel. Some workers get special gloves. Others wear earplugs. But no company we know of issues comfortable shoes or gives its employees free foot massages to help prevent 25 percent of all industrial accidents, the ones the U.S. Department of Labor says are directly related to *fatigued feet*. And foot problems at work are only the tip (or toe) of the iceberg. With 26 delicate bones and the burden of bearing your entire body weight at every step, even nonunion feet can go on strike.

Podiatrists say that people who stand for several hours at a time have it worse than people who move around. "Standing involves 100 percent of foot use, while walking requires only about 40 percent," says California foot specialist Dennis Augustine, D.P.M. "When you walk, your feet alternate the load, with one foot getting a rest half of the time. But when you stand, the load is constant." To ease the strain of all-day standing, keep your feet as active as possible, he says. Wiggle 'em, rock 'em, roll 'em—or even get one of those rubber doormats with all the little rubber nipples to stand on. They not only cushion, they also provide exercise as your feet try to adjust to the mat's "variable terrain."

This is not to say that people on the move have perfect feet, with no aches and pains. Being constantly on the go means that your feet can suffer a great deal of abuse—particularly if you often wear shoes that constrict or bind. But if you're moving around, your feet also get a lot of *use*, which leads to better blood circulation. "Feet are at the remote end of your circulatory system," podiatrist Timothy P. Shea, D.P.M., author of *The Over Easy Foot Care Book*, explains. "They must work hard to pump blood back to the heart." Dr. Shea believes people would have fewer foot problems if they exercised throughout life. "Exercise keeps the muscles, tendons and ligaments of the foot flexible, and flexible feet make it easier to keep exercising." Walking is one of the best things you can do to prevent aching feet, he adds.

But you could be doing your feet a disservice (and could be headed for some hefty medical bills) if you exercise your feet in the wrong shoes. Dr. Augustine says that a good shoe is of "utmost importance"—for exercise and for everyday wear. He recommends looking for these key elements: good support, good cushioning, a wide toe-box and a low heel. Avoid plastic and rubber shoes, too, since they trap moisture and can promote infection.

If you must wear high heels, says Dr. Shea, try to limit the height to 2 inches. "Shoes with heels over 2 inches high put excess pressure on the front of your foot. They can cause calluses and bursitis [swelling of the sacs next to the joints on the feet] as well as back problems."

High heels with pointed toes frequently are the culprits behind bunions, say foot experts. Bunions develop when the big toe is forced toward the other toes, exposing the outer joint to friction against the shoe. Not only are bunions unsightly, they're painful, too. But Walter H. O. Bohne, M.D., of the Hospital for Special Surgery in New York City, has a tip to help avoid and relieve bunions: "Ideally, you should change your shoes once a day. At home, you might want to wear *zori*, Japanese

How to Doctor an Ingrown Toenail

Save some money and a visit to the foot doctor with this no-surgery method for giving ingrown toenails the boot. It comes from Harold Fishman, M.D., a Los Angeles-based dermatologist who says it works in 80 percent of all cases. First, Dr. Fishman advises, push the skin away from the nail with a piece of cotton rolled to twice the thickness of a candle wick. Place the cotton between the skin and the nail, add iodine and wrap the toe with gauze and tape. Eventually, a sharp and spiky nail will grow, which can be filed off with an emery board. Add a drop of iodine every day and change the wick once a week. Give the toe 3 to 6 weeks to heal.

reed-soled shoes with a thong between the toes. They help straighten out the big toe, and the reed soles give the feet something to grip for exercise."

TLC FOR YOUR FEET

The feet like tender loving care, says Dr. Augustine. He suggests massaging your feet with lanolin, cocoa butter, baby oil or even rubbing alcohol. End with a foot soak using warm water and Epsom salts.

Dry your feet thoroughly and powder them after bathing, advises Dr. Shea, to protect against developing painful fungal infections. Also, clip your toenails straight across so they don't become ingrown. "But never do bathroom surgery," he cautions. "It's too easy to cut normal tissue when you use razor blades to trim hard tissue."

For mildly irritating corns, Dr. Shea recommends placing a thin strip of moleskin on the toe to reduce friction from the shoe. For soft corns (usually the corns between the toes that stay soft because they are kept moist), use lamb's wool between the toes to separate them and reduce moisture.

For calluses, says Dr. Augustine, buy a pumice stone (available at drugstores) and gently rub off deadened skin in the bath or shower.

For heel spurs, a condition caused by calcium deposits on the bone itself, insert heel pads into the shoe. Made of felt or sponge rubber, heel pads work well when you cut holes in the material to fit under the painful areas.

For sore arches, commercially produced arch supports can be a boon. But if they don't help, you may want to see a specialist to be fitted for professionally custom-designed orthotics to aid your feet.

For all-around healthy feet, inspect your feet daily. "Take the time to run your hands over the soles of your feet, and really look at them," says Dr. Bohne. Your feet will appreciate the care.

Let a Foot Map Guide You to Better Health

There's a healing art that deals primarily with the feet—foot reflexology. By stimulating specific points on the feet, say reflexologists, the body is encouraged to heal itself. "On the foot is a mini-map of the body," says Laura Norman, a certified reflexologist from New York City. "Certain points correspond to specific parts of the body, acting like electrical hotlines to distant tissues and systems. Obviously, reflexology does wonders to relieve aching feet," she continues, "but it can also relieve many stress-related disorders such as headaches and backaches. Basically, it relaxes the entire body." You can practice it on yourself and others, she says, mainly by bending the thumb and walking it forward, pressing into the reflex areas pictured here. Hold onto the feet with your fingers for leverage.

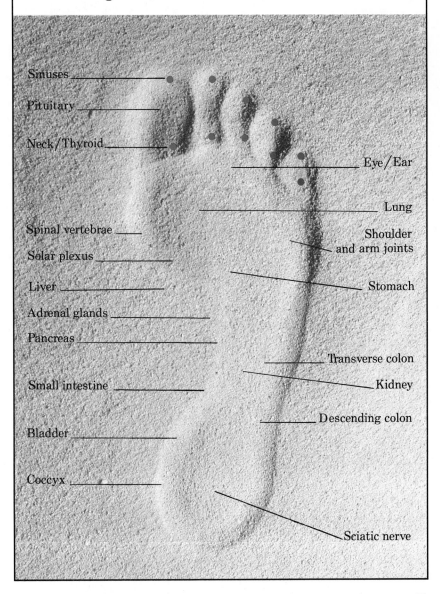

Sinuses
Pituitary
Neck/Thyroid
Eye/Ear
Lung
Spinal vertebrae
Shoulder and arm joints
Solar plexus
Stomach
Liver
Adrenal glands
Pancreas
Transverse colon
Kidney
Small intestine
Descending colon
Bladder
Coccyx
Sciatic nerve

Muscle and Menstrual Cramps

Muscle cramps attack when an already shortened muscle is contracted still further. The muscle gets tighter and tighter until it hardens into a spasmodic mass and finally sends a distress signal to the brain: Do something! It hurts!

Some of the most common cramps affect *skeletal* muscles, such as those in the feet, legs and abdomen. Skeletal muscles are under voluntary control, and they work in pairs. When one relaxes, another contracts. To see for yourself how this works, bend one arm at the elbow. The muscles on the inside of your arm contract—shorten—to set the arm in motion. But at the same time, the muscles along the outer edge of your arm elongate, or relax.

You can put this pairing system to work to your advantage when you need to unknot cramped skeletal muscles: Your aim is to extend, or relax, the pained muscle. How? One way is to contract the muscle that works *in opposition* to the cramped muscle.

This is a principle you've probably put to work already, if you have ever had a leg cramp sneak up on you at night. It's likely you got out of bed and tried "walking it out," which serves to stretch the muscle causing all the trouble.

Nocturnal leg cramps attack seemingly out of the blue, unlike cramps that you get after vigorous exercise or muscle strain. They usually affect the calf muscle or the sole of the foot; either can be exquisitely painful.

STAND UP FOR YOURSELF

Considering the way some people sleep, it's no wonder legs cramp up at night, says Israel H. Weiner, M.D., of the department of neurological surgery at the University of Maryland School of Medicine. Dr. Weiner points out that heavy, tight bed covers tend to place the feet in the "passive plantar flexed position" —which means that the toes and top of the foot stretch downward. People who sleep on their stomach also inadvertently place their feet in this position. As you can easily see, that means the opposing muscles along the sole of the foot and the calf are forcibly shortened. Nerve impulses sent to the spinal column keep telling those muscles to contract in response to the continuous stretched position of the top of the feet. The nerve impulses keep firing this message long after it's physiologically comfortable for the contracting muscle. It contracts and contracts and . . . suddenly the muscle is a hard wad of pain, and *finally* the spinal column receives signals of pain.

Here's how to get rid of that cramp—fast.

1. Stand up and stretch the muscle. Then walk around for a few minutes.

2. If standing is too painful,

A blanket support isn't very cozy-looking, but it will keep bed covers from weighing down the tops of your feet, reducing your chances of getting a foot or leg cramp. (See the Buyer's Guide on page 162.)

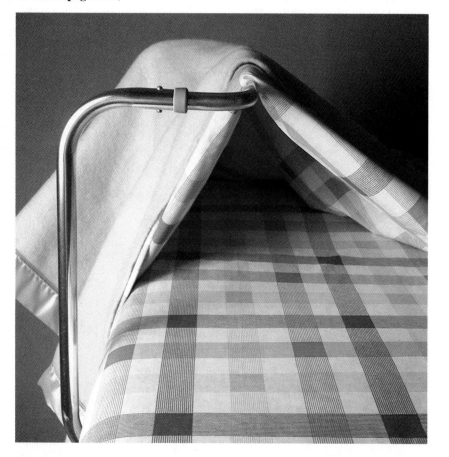

26

massage the knotted muscle, kneading it into submission. You may even want to try a warm cloth to relax the muscle, but relax it must, in order for you to gain relief.

3. When you go back to bed, says Dr. Weiner, place a pillow against the soles of your feet to keep them from assuming the passive plantar position. Keep the bed covers loose; you may even want to purchase a blanket support, such as the one shown on the opposite page, to hold the covers up. And if you like sleeping on your stomach, let your feet extend over the edge of the mattress "to maintain a more neutral foot position," he advises.

AN EXERCISE TO PREVENT CRAMPS

Drug therapy—in the form of muscle relaxants—is "frequently recommended" for preventing leg cramps at night, says Dr. Weiner, but, he adds, "it is seldom necessary or justified." Instead there is an exercise you can do daily to stretch the calf muscles. Designed by H. W. Daniell, M.D., who claims it's effective in half of his patients, it requires no more equipment than a bare wall. Stand barefoot about a yard away from the wall and lean forward, keeping your heels on the floor. Support your weight against the wall with your hands. Hold this position for 10 seconds. Then push back to the starting position, count to 5 and repeat the exercise.

"Stretching out the calf that way helps tone the muscle," says Mary Jane Wolbers, a dance educator and professor at East Stroudsburg University in Pennsylvania. "Walking around in bare feet or wearing flat shoes for a period of time every day will help, too. Women who wear high-heeled shoes all their lives will eventually find that their Achilles tendon (in the back of the heel) has

been permanently shortened, forcing the calf muscle into a constant state of contraction and predisposing it to cramping. The calf muscle loses its ability to relax properly. In fact, some women can never go without heels—they even wear slippers with heels—because it's too painful to stand flat."

In addition, regular exercise such as walking will help stretch the calf muscle, and improve circulation in the legs and feet.

Blood circulation plays a central role in muscle health and function. Blood supplies energy, fresh oxygen and essential nutrients to the muscle tissues. But all the exercise in the world won't improve circulation if you aren't feeding the blood with nutrients it demands.

TWO NUTRIENTS THAT CAN HELP BANISH CRAMPS

One of the nutrients doctors have found useful in treating cramps is vitamin E.

An Australian physician, L. Lotzof, M.D., has reported, "I have now tried vitamin E with remarkable success on approximately 50 patients suffering from muscular cramp . . . and have found that approximately 300 milligrams (447 I.U.) taken daily was sufficient to control most cramping." (This amount of vitamin E should be taken only with your doctor's okay.)

But vitamin E isn't the only aid for cramping of skeletal muscles. Calcium is also known to abolish the problem, because the muscles need calcium in order to relax and lengthen. Medical reports of its value go back a long way: "There is a time-honored belief that calcium metabolism has something to do with [cramps], and indeed calcium lactate or gluconate, vitamin D and a glass of milk on retiring often seem to work," according to the *British Medical Journal*.

Cramping Your Freestyle

Is there really a stomach cramp monster that sniffs out full-bellied swimmers? Jane Katz, Ed.D., an aquatics specialist, says that while muscle cramps may bother you if you swim too soon after eating a full meal, these cramps won't be in your stomach. You could suffer abdominal *discomfort* because of the increased workload on the digestive system, however.

Dr. Katz says that the best time to swim is 3 to 4 hours after a full meal. And what you eat is as important as when you eat. Avoid high-protein, high-fat foods: They take too long to digest. Instead, have something high in complex carbohydrates. "If you swim during lunch hour," says Dr. Katz, "instead of a doughnut at your 10 A.M. coffee break, eat a piece of fruit. By noon, your blood sugar levels will be just about right."

Ralph Smiley, M.D., of the Environmental Control Unit at Brookhaven Hospital in Dallas, Texas, says that cramping is commonly associated with calcium deficiency. "We make sure all our patients with cramps are getting enough calcium," he says.

It's great to know that nocturnal leg cramps need not forever thwart your chances of getting a good night's sleep. But what about cramps that come on after you've lifted something too heavy, or cramps brought on by too-strenuous exercise—or just ordinary side stitches that double you up while you're out jogging?

A Dancer's Trick for Leg Cramps

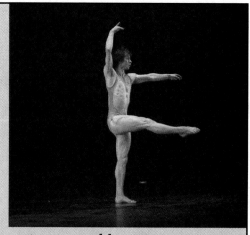

Any time a dancer goes up on pointe, or extends a graceful leg straight out into space, the calf muscles and other muscles along the back of the legs contract—and keep contracting for minutes at a time. That can mean tight muscles, which not only compromise performance but lead to excruciating cramps as well. So to increase flexibility, says E. C. Frederick, Ph.D., director of research at Nike, a dancer "will tense the muscles on the front of the legs. The reason: Increased tension in one group of muscles causes the opposite muscles to relax."

You can put this trick into action to relax leg cramps, says dance education specialist Mary Jane Wolbers. She says to stand barefoot and flex the front of your foot as hard as you can, keeping your heels on the floor. Or you can stand on a stair with your heels hanging off the edge. "It's even better than simple flexing exercises," she says, "because you've added the weight of your body to the stretch."

NO MORE EXERCISE CRAMPS

The best way to get rid of exercise-induced cramps is to avoid getting them in the first place. Exercise is important, but so is treating your muscles kindly: The human body simply wasn't designed to bench-press pianos.

Whatever you do, avoid *over*doing it. Even Olympic athletes are subject to muscle cramping, particularly as they push their muscles to the limit. What happens is that the muscles grow swollen and tight from all the activity, and it becomes more and more difficult for the blood and lymph to pass freely to the muscles. Stores of glycogen (our body's main energy source) drop and the muscle dehydrates. Waste products that are normally carried off by these fluids— especially lactic acid—build up. Starved for oxygen and glutted with lactic acid, the muscle cannot perform well and goes into spasm.

Massage is one good way to calm the throbbing muscle, as it increases blood and lymph flow and helps wring out lactic acid. But a gentle warmup and stretching well *after* any activity may preclude the need for massage altogether (see chapter 4). Also, a 5-minute walk before and after running will limber up stiffened muscles.

Budd Coates, a corporate fitness director and world-class marathon athlete, says that breathing properly is particularly crucial for people plagued with side stitches.

Stitches occur in the diaphragm, a muscle under the ribcage. And breathing from the diaphragm, says Coates, makes you less susceptible to stitches. Should you get a stitch, "change your breathing pattern from deep rhythmic breathing to shallow quick breathing, or vice versa," he says.

One last tip for cramping that hits after a workout: It may be related to heat and dehydration. Unless you're bicycling across the desert, though, salt tablets aren't what's called for—water and other fluids are.

MONTHLY CRAMPS

Some of the most common cramps of all are menstrual cramps, whether they're mild twinges or the debilitating, wrenching pain of dysmenorrhea.

The uterine muscles, which are smooth muscles and therefore not under voluntary control, contract in waves (for some women, *tidal* waves), usually during the beginning of the period.

The culprits behind the pain appear to be hormonelike substances called prostaglandins, which are secreted in the fluid of the uterine lining. The menstrual fluid of women who suffer severe dysmenorrhea contains abnormally high amounts of these prostaglandins. When the prostaglandins are produced in excess, the uterus contracts, squeezing so hard that oxygen supply to the blood vessels is cut off. The result: pain. Some prostaglandins even escape into the bloodstream, where they affect other smooth muscles like the intestines, causing the diarrhea that's common early in a woman's period.

If your cramps are very bothersome, an obvious solution is to have your doctor prescribe a prostaglandin-inhibiting drug. Aspirin, too, is an antiprostaglandin that helps some women. Taken once a month, these drugs rarely cause any worrisome side effects and are very effective.

There are some natural nondrug comfort measures, too, that you can take to quell menstrual cramps. Malissa Martin, an athletic trainer from the University of South Carolina, Columbia, uses acupressure to relieve menstrual cramps in athletes. In one study, she found it helped 60 percent of her athletic charges. You can have someone locate the effective pressure point by first bending your head to your chest, she says. Then, starting from the bump located at the base of your neck, have your partner count down 15 more bumps to the third lumbar vertebra. About ¾ inch to 1½ inches to the right of that point, there

should be a sensitive area. That's where your partner should begin pressing down lightly and then around in circles once the pain starts to let up. In 2 to 10 minutes, you should feel much better.

Another acupressure point for menstrual pain is on the inner ankle. To find it, cradle one foot in your lap. Find a tender spot about midway between the ankle bone and the Achilles tendon and apply gentle pressure with the thumb.

If you're at home—or even at the office—don't underestimate the healing power of a good old-fashioned hot water bottle. Many women report that warmth against the abdomen helps banish cramps, whether they're clutching a hot water bottle, a pile of covers or a pillow.

And with all the hoopla and general attention on PMS (premenstrual syndrome), it's not surprising that doctors have now come up with nutritional supplement combinations that may ease uterine cramping. Alan Gaby, M.D., a nutritional therapist in Baltimore, says that vitamin B_6 (no more than 50 milligrams per day) and magnesium are the foundations of a menstrual cramp formula he gives his patients. Other nutrients in his formula are calcium, zinc and essential fatty acids.

"It's a very good combination," Dr. Gaby says, "although we're not positive exactly why all these things work together so well. But we believe it's related to the whole prostaglandin system."

Finally, you may have heard that exercise helps cramping. But if your cramps are the kind that feel as though you're still being punished for Eve's mistake, you know that running around the block would be even more punishment. Actually, some movement *can* ease cramps, but it's the gentle, yoga-based exercise that helps—often referred to as postures rather than out-and-out exercise. The exercises on pages 30 and 31 should bring quick, soothing relief.

Easing Menstrual Cramps

When menstrual cramps become unbearable, your natural instinct is to double over or curl up on your side. So you've probably discovered that the fetal position is a fine remedy for the pain that you're feeling. These exercises adapt the natural healing power of that position to help when the going gets rough.

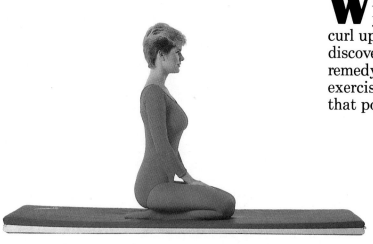

1 Choose a quiet, preferably carpeted, spot. Kneel on the floor, knees together, sitting back on your heels with the tops of your feet flat on the floor.

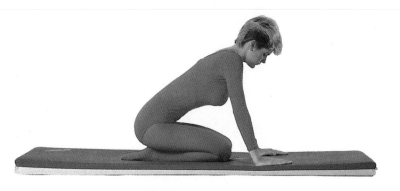

2 Slowly bend forward, sliding your arms and hands—palms flat—straight out in front of you until your back is rounded and your chest touches your legs.

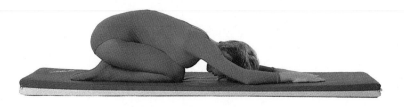

3 Stretch out and touch your forehead to the floor. Hold this position as long as you like, breathing normally, with your eyes closed.

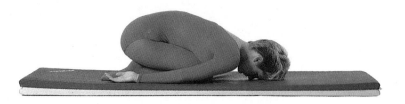

4 When you feel relaxed, open your eyes and pull your arms straight back along your sides, bringing them to rest with the palms up.

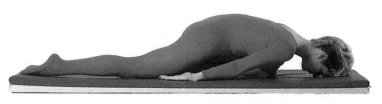

5 Slide your left leg straight back as far as it will go. Then draw it back under the abdomen. Repeat at your own pace, alternating legs.

6 Next, slowly return to the original crouched position. Holding your knees to your chest, roll over onto your back.

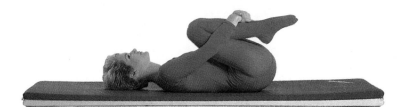

7 Slowly lower your legs into a bent-knee position until your feet are flat on the floor, about a foot away from your buttocks. Relax your arms at your sides, palms down.

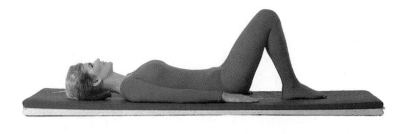

8 Tighten your stomach muscles and lift your hips off the floor in a "bridge" so that your trunk and legs form a straight line to the knees.

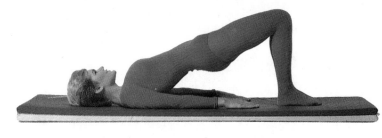

9 Slowly lower your hips and back to the floor, and when you are fully down, push down toward the floor with the small of your back. (Just to make sure you're working the right area, place one hand under the arch of your back and try to press your back against your hand.)

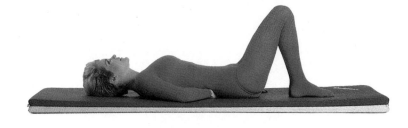

10 Release and return to your original position. Relax, breathe slowly and steadily. When you are ready, repeat the sequence at your own pace.

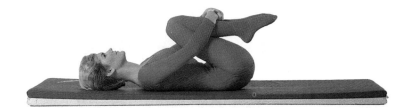

Backaches

It's the playoff of the 1984 United States Open championship—18 extra holes that will decide the winner of golf's most prized title. On the second hole, Fuzzy Zoeller sinks a 68-foot putt for a birdie—and goes on to sink his opponent by eight strokes. But Zoeller had started competing before he ever teed off.

Two hours before the match began, he put on a beltlike device that sent gentle waves of electric current into his lower back. You see, he has a handicap that doesn't show up on his scorecard, a problem that's more painful than a double bogey—a bad back.

Zoeller hurt his back playing high school basketball. For the rest of us (only one out of every five people is completely free of back pain, according to one estimate), it could have been the way we lifted the baby out of the crib. Or the car accident that jolted our head and neck like a punching bag. Or the desk job that freezes us into a slouch for 8 hours a day. In fact, it seems that almost anything can cause a bad back—and that nothing short of a spinal transplant can cure it.

But a back isn't like food left out on the counter—it doesn't go bad just because it's there. There are easy, effective ways to make a bad back behave—or keep a good one at its best.

That's the opinion of Jerome M. Cotler, M.D., a professor of orthopedic surgery at Jefferson Medical College in Philadelphia. "The best ways to reduce your risk of back injuries or problems," he says, "are to exercise regularly, avoid remaining in fixed positions for long periods of time, avoid severe twists and turns and keep your weight down."

He maintains that back problems requiring traction, surgery and other radical measures of treatment are the rare exceptions, not the rule, affecting only around 2 percent of all back pain sufferers. That jibes with what other back experts say: The vast majority of backaches are due to muscle strain, which can be treated with simple, at-home methods, rather than by a pinched nerve or a slipped disk, which need a doctor's trained eye and advice.

"Slipped disks are not quite as common as you might think," says Hans Kraus, M.D., author of *Backaches, Stress and Tension.* "Many people who think they're suffering from disk trouble actually are victims of muscle strain in the

Just Hangin' Around

Maybe bats are smarter than we thought. According to Somerset, New Jersey, chiropractor Fred Kingsbury, D.C., their habit of hanging upside-down is a very good one—so good, in fact, that he uses it to treat a variety of back problems.

Dr. Kingsbury said that one of the main benefits of hanging upside-down, or inversion therapy, is that it takes the pressure off your back by reversing the pull of gravity.

But Dr. Kingsbury stresses that inversion therapy is *not* for people who have certain conditions, including high blood pressure, glaucoma, acute strains or fractures. And you should *always* have professional guidance before you begin.

Some inversion systems are more therapeutic than others. Dr. Kingsbury recommends the Orthopod (pictured here), because it "doesn't put any strain on the ankles, knees or hips."

back, and this condition can be corrected through exercise instead of surgery."

In fact, exercise rates as the single most important thing you can do to protect your back. Since muscle spasms are at the root of back pain, it makes sense to keep the muscles toned, well stretched, well relaxed and in all-around good shape.

"When muscles are weak through lack of exercise," says Dr. Kraus, "they can't do their share of keeping the body erect, and too much strain falls on the bones and ligaments of your spine."

Exercise is doubly important for aging backs, says Willibald Nagler, M.D., of New York Hospital.

"Muscles tend to deteriorate with age for most people because they lead sedentary lives," says Dr. Nagler. "Add to that the usual changes that occur in our spine as we get older. We tend to get a little shorter from bone shrinkage, there's a thinning of the disks and the spine often develops arthritic spurs. But the muscular insufficiencies of the back, stomach and hips usually cause the most pain and immobility. That's why increasing the strength and flexibility of those muscles almost always brings relief."

The best exercises to do for your back involve strengthening the muscles of the abdomen, not the back muscles themselves. That's because the abdominals take the weight off our back and help brace the spine—sort of like guy wires holding a pole in place. (See pages 34 and 35 for exercises specifically designed to ease backache and prevent trouble from recurring.)

But movement is a mixed blessing. While the rhythmic, steady throb of exercise can tone and strengthen back muscles, sudden or unusual motions can strain muscles so that they go into self-protecting spasms— the body's last-ditch effort to keep the injured areas rigid and still.

Muscular spasms are rarely set off by accident, explains Dr. Nagler. "When your back 'goes out,' it's more than likely from an activity your body isn't used to doing. And

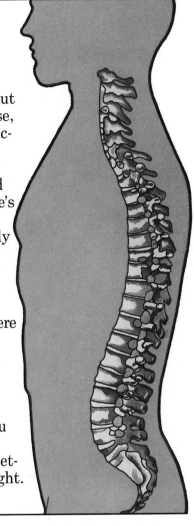

Is a Chiropractor for You?

You don't often hear jokes about chiropractors on the golf course, or the cry, "Is there a chiropractor in the house?" But this healing profession (the name means "done by hand"), based largely on theories of the spine's relationship to health, just keeps on growing. It has nearly doubled in the last 15 years.

Why? According to one study of people with back problems, patients felt more welcomed by chiropractors, were more satisfied with the treatment they received and were able to return to work sooner than others who saw M.D.'s.

So if you have a back problem—particularly one you think is muscle- or skeleton-related—you might consider letting a chiropractor set it straight.

it's not necessarily a high-energy-expenditure activity, either, like shoveling snow all day. Often just reaching for something, unprepared, causes the muscles to tighten up. Moving a piece of furniture or yanking luggage from a conveyor belt at the airport can leave you instantly paralyzed with pain if you're susceptible."

So what can you do about those crisis times when your back "goes out" or just hurts like the devil? Here are some suggestions from some top back experts.

R_x FOR BACK PAIN

Rest in Bed. According to Dr. Cotler, bed rest is the mainstay of

(continued on page 36)

Daily Back Relief

Practice these exercises daily to help relieve back pain. The leg slide, arm exercise and seat relaxer will calm tense muscles. The others will increase muscle flexibility. To start, wear comfortable clothes and socks (but no shoes). To prevent injuries, exercise on a mat or carpet, not a soft mattress or a hard floor.

Half Sit-Up

Lie on your back, with your knees bent and arms at your sides. Inhale deeply, then exhale slowly through your mouth as you come to a half sit-up position. Bring your fingertips to the tops of your knees, then lower your trunk and uncurl slowly. Relax. Repeat twice.

Leg Slide

Lie flat on your back and close your eyes. Place your arms at your sides and bend your knees. Take a deep breath and exhale slowly through your mouth. Then slide one leg forward on the mat until it is fully extended. Slide back to the bent-knee position. Repeat with the other leg. Take another breath. Exhale slowly. Clench both fists and then relax them.

Seat Relaxer

Lie on your stomach and rest your forehead on your hands. Point your toes inward. Take a deep breath and exhale slowly through your mouth. Tighten your buttocks. Hold for 2 seconds and then let go. Repeat twice.

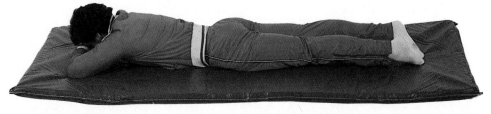

Hamstring Stretch

Lie on your back, with your arms at your sides and knees bent. Bring one knee up toward your chest. Then unfold the leg toward the ceiling and lock your knee, pointing your toes up. Keep the leg straight and lower it to the mat. Slide the leg back to the bent-knee position and relax. Repeat with the other leg.

Arm Exercise

Lying on your back, bend one arm up at the elbow. Then let it drop easily to the mat. Repeat with the other arm. Take a deep breath and exhale slowly through your mouth.

Fetal Position

Turn on your side, with your eyes closed, knees bent, and your head on your arm. Place the other arm in front of you or on your hip. Breathe deeply and exhale slowly through your mouth. Slide your upper leg toward your shoulder along the floor, then straighten it. Slide it back to the fetal position. Repeat twice on this side, then switch sides.

Eight Ways to Bid a Backache Goodnight

- Choose a firm mattress. An "orthopedic" hard bed, a 10-inch-deep water bed or mattress pads of pure wool with dense, tufted, fleecy pile will offer superior sleeping comfort.
- Lie on your side and draw one or both of your knees up toward your chin.
- Keep your arms relaxed at your sides rather than over your head.
- Don't use a high pillow; it can lead to neck and back cramping.
- Avoid foam rubber pillows. Opt for fiber-fill or down instead.
- Wear loose-fitting night-clothes.
- When you lie on your back, place a pillow under your knees to relieve pressure.
- If you must sleep on your stomach, raise one arm and leg to minimize strain on your neck or place a pillow under your hips.

treatment, and often all that is needed to ease most backaches.

Apply Ice Packs. When a patient shows up on Dr. Nagler's doorstep with acute muscle spasms, "we lay the patient down and put an ice pack right where the spasm is. After the painful area is numb," he continues, "we apply some electrical stimulation, which induces normal contraction and relaxation of the muscle." Once the pain has subsided, Dr. Nagler introduces simple limbering-up exercises.

Consider Your Back in All Activities of Daily Living. That's the advice of Hamilton Hall, M.D., author of *The Back Doctor.* Don't sit for long periods of time, for instance. Sitting can create a greater load on your spine than standing. When lifting, pass work on to the legs. And remember: "The most hazardous lifts are the ones for which you are unprepared." Also, never twist and lift at the same time.

Another back specialist adds that rolling out of bed is a good way to be nice to your back. She explains that most people don't roll out of bed; they sit up, putting strain on the back. Ideally, she says, you should do some stretching before getting up, then roll to the edge of the bed, place your feet on the floor and use your arms to push yourself up.

But the activities of daily living can also include special events—little tricks you can use to keep your back in line. Here's the story of a woman with back pain who was going to throw in the towel—until she used it in an unusual way.

A TOWEL TO THE RESCUE

"What am I going to do?" moaned Margaret. It had taken two weeks of rest for her back to recover from a long bus ride—from Tulsa, Oklahoma,

to Cape Cod, Massachusetts—and now it was time to board the bus back to Tulsa. She dreaded the journey, wincing as she remembered the stabbing pains in her lower back that had kept her from fully enjoying this vacation with friends. She was just beginning to feel good again and knew that the uncomfortable bus seat, plus bumping around for long hours on end, spelled trouble. And pain.

Her friend sympathized. "I have a friend who's a physical therapist," she told Margaret. "He lives in another state, but let's give him a call anyway and see if he has anything to say that might help."

The therapist *did* have something to say. "Very simple. Tell your friend to roll up a towel and place it in the seat directly behind the small of her back. It'll support that area of her back."

Margaret called once she'd arrived home, to say that it was a safe and interesting trip. "And tell your friend that I feel fantastic. The towel really worked! In fact, I'm using one at my desk now, too."

Thanks to a rolled-up piece of cloth, strategically placed, Margaret was able to spare herself a great deal of pain and inconvenience.

If you've got a bum back, you've probably discovered a few tricks for yourself. Some people take a hot shower every morning, aiming a massage shower head toward sore spots or areas on the back that take a lot of tension during the day. Other people disdain the usual feather pillows in favor of cervical pillows that are designed to hold the upper spine during sleep.

Whatever you do for your back, and no matter who you go to for back pain—be it a doctor, a physical therapist or a chiropractor—remember that early warning signs of pain should not be ignored. If healthy back practices are part of your daily life, however, you can save yourself from feeling those twinges at all.

How to Give a Great Backrub

"Ummmm," "Ahhhhh," or maybe even "Zzzzzz." Those are the sounds of a wonderful massage, one of life's most soothing experiences—whether your tension comes from sitting rigidly at a desk or from laboring on the loading docks.

And giving a massage can be just as rewarding and relaxing as getting one. Almost all of us already soothe, comfort and communicate by touch. But just a few minutes given to learning some simple skills can transform your amateur ability into Olympic-level talent. Here are some key pointers on massaging the back and shoulders, one of tension's favorite tightening spots.

Choose a comfortable place where you and your partner will be undisturbed. Use a padded table or floor; a bed doesn't provide proper support. Using oil is highly recommended. Any light vegetable oil will do; almond is nice.

Relax yourself first. Get calm. Concentrate on the present moment. Starting from a position behind your partner's head, rub downward from the shoulders with your hands shaped into V's and your thumbs pressing alongside the spine, but not on the spine itself. Return your hands up the sides. Repeat this maneuver several times. Throughout the massage, keep one or both hands on your partner.

Again, working down from the shoulders with your hands in the same V position, use your thumbs to make small, firm circles on the muscles alongside the spine.

To get at ultra-tense hidden muscles, gently lift your partner's arm and place that hand behind the waist. Supporting your partner's elbow with one hand, use your other hand to rub the area under the shoulder blade.

For a relaxing shoulder rub, support the shoulder from underneath with one hand as you gently knead the muscles on top with the other. Now—prepare yourself for profuse compliments and thank-you's.

Tools That Work to Save Your Back

Are the daily activities that used to be a breeze now more difficult because of your aching back? Rather than giving up, why not try to outwit your back troubles with these handy tools—specially designed with your back in mind—that make yard work and desk work a breeze. (See the Buyer's Guide on page 162 for catalog and ordering information.)

Easy Shovel and Rake

The handles of these tools are bent, so your back won't be. This design puts the pressure right on the shovel or rake head, so you get the job done without having to lean over and push. This takes a lot of strain off your back. These tools work wonderfully on snowy sidewalks and leaf-cluttered lawns.

Balans Chair

It's nearly impossible to have poor posture when you sit on a Balans chair. The chairs are also remarkably comfortable at work or home because they let your back maintain its natural curves, with your head straight above your tailbone, just as nature intended.

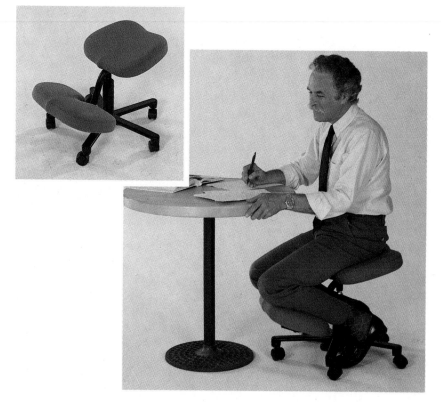

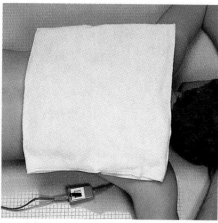

Moist Heat

This heating pad draws its own moisture from the air, keeps an even temperature and is a nice alternative to dripping towels that start out scalding but soon become cold and clammy.

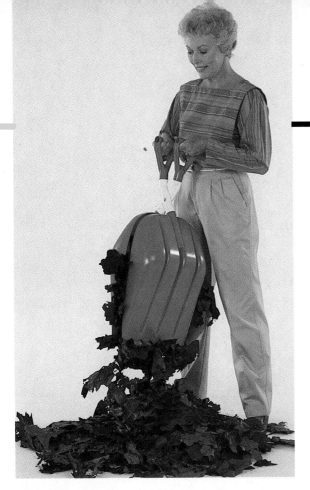

Big Scoop

Bending to the ground to pick up leaves, compost or sand becomes a distant memory when you have Lawn Claws. They hold a big load, and all you have to do is squeeze the handles and lift with your arms. Makes quick work of jobs that people with aching backs often try to avoid.

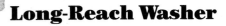

Long-Reach Washer

No more ladders or painful stretching needed when you use this handy window washer and wall scrubber with a high-pressure hose tip.

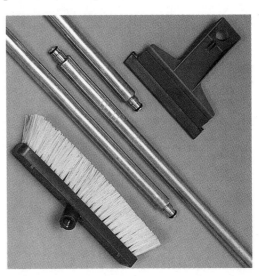

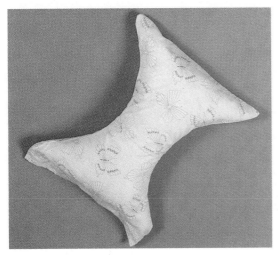

Neck Support

This pillow is just the right shape to stave off stiff necks, and back and shoulder pain. It supports your head and neck as it relieves strain on your spine.

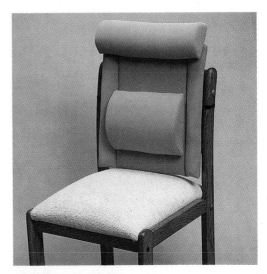

Adjustable Back Support

Two adjustable pads, one for the lower back and one for the shoulder area, make this a custom cushion. Designed by an orthopedist to provide optimum comfort and support, the cushion fits any chair.

3

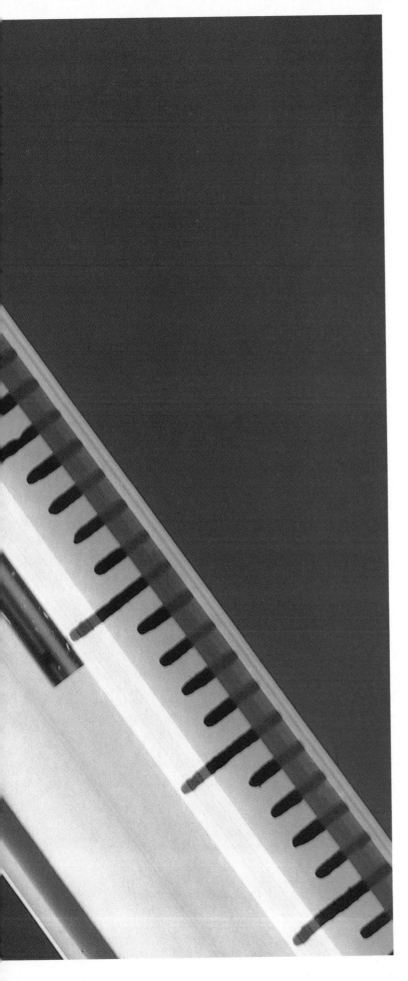

Beating the Bug

The best home treatments for infections of all kinds.

Feeling too hot? Too cold? Tired? Itchy? Out of sorts? Could be that you're coming down with whatever is going around.

Even if you're normally in the pink of health, doing everything you can to stay fit and strong, sooner or later you're bound to fall prey to one bug or another. Short of staying in permanent quarantine, it's hardly possible to isolate yourself from the invisible organisms all around us. Our air, water and food, as well as every surface in our surroundings—and our bodies—teem with countless numbers of these microorganisms. Some of them are congenial or even necessary to our body's ecosystems; others threaten it.

Normally, our body deflects the troublesome organisms—in fact, we're usually oblivious to them until we lose a battle with one and succumb to illness.

These hostile microbes can be divided into several basic categories. *Bacteria* are small, single-celled organisms that wreak havoc by producing toxins in our system or by rousing the body's defenses, causing swelling, pus or inflammation. *Viruses* are so small they can be seen only with an electron microscope. They actually enter and take over cell nuclei, eventually destroying them. *Fungi* are plantlike organisms that multiply on the surface layer of the skin. Still other organisms are intermediate; they have some of the physical properties of bacteria but act like viruses.

Our best protection against these bugs is to fortify our immune system. Failing that, we must rely on treatments to kill the invaders or at least ease the painful symptoms as our bodies wage war.

The next time you or someone in your family picks up a bug, take comfort. In this chapter, we'll tell you about the most effective remedies for some of these contagious critters, from colds and flu to athlete's foot, pinkeye and venereal infections.

Colds and Flu

The common cold is like the unwanted relative in our lives; a definite nuisance we wearily come to expect at the same time each year. It leaves only when it's good and ready, despite all efforts to shoo it away.

Both colds and a similar but more serious infection—the flu—attack a critical pathway in our bodies, the upper respiratory system. This 16-inch tract of bones, muscles and cartilage, connected by tubes and flaps, is intricate and complex—and frail at times, especially if we fail to safeguard it.

Chills and Colds: A Myth That Melts

"Don't get chilled—you'll catch pneumonia," we've all heard Mom warn. But in this instance, Mom's instincts simply haven't been backed by scientific fact. Getting a chill has nothing to do with catching a cold, a finding that several studies can back up, according to John Mills, M.D., chief of the division of infectious diseases at San Francisco General Hospital Medical Center. Mills noted that in one study, volunteers were subjected to particularly Draconian treatment to find out whether getting chilled causes a cold. Some volunteers stood naked in 60-degree temperatures for 4 hours, while others stood clothed in 10-degree temperatures for 2 hours. The two groups were then exposed to cold viruses. They came down with upper respiratory infections at the same rates. There was no difference in the severity of their colds, researchers found. "Frequent changes in the weather possibly lower your resistance to colds when you don't dress properly for the weather, but they don't cause colds," says Lois Hoskins, R.N., an assistant professor of medical-surgical nursing at the Catholic University of America School of Nursing, Washington, D.C. In fact, scientists at the South Pole, who must constantly contend with the elements, prove that colds have more to do with viruses than with weather. Despite the fact that temperatures regularly dive to 100 degrees below zero there, the scientists almost never catch colds.

TELLING THEM APART

Although colds and flu are often mistaken for one another because they share many of the same symptoms, there are several ways to tell them apart. Flu almost always begins suddenly, with a fever of at least 100°, unlike colds, which gather momentum slowly. Flu is usually marked by a generally weak, headachy feeling; chills; wide-spread muscle aches; fever; watery, sore eyes and a dry, hacking cough. The incubation period, from the time of exposure to the full bloom of symptoms, is usually 24 to 48 hours. Flu viruses generally strike lots of people at the same time. If nobody around you has the flu, it's unlikely that's what you've got.

While colds don't usually knock you down for the count, they can be ornery and persistent and cause plenty of discomfort. Your head can feel like a cinderblock; your nose, red and raw, exudes a constant, running stream and you can sneeze and cough to the point of exhaustion.

Fortunately, no one has to be sentenced to a life term of colds and viral afflictions every time the seasons change. You can build up your own system to fend them off.

THE COLD FACTS

The first step is knowing what causes colds and the flu. First, damp, chill weather won't make you catch a cold, although it may lower your resistance to germs. Actually, colds are usually caught from other people with colds—often before they develop active symptoms. When they sneeze, cough, yawn or even talk, they send tiny virus-laden droplets into the air. But that's not the most common way of catching a cold. Rather than saying you "caught" a cold, you might start saying you were *handed* a cold, since hands that squelched a cough or sneeze, then touched a doorknob or a piece of paper, are the most common media for transmitting a cold. If you touch an infected hand or object, then rub your eyes or nose—bing—you've got a cold, too. So if you're around someone with a cold, it's advisable to keep your hands away from your nose and eyes, the body's most common receiving points for such germs.

Many folks blame their sniffles on the cold outside, but the culprit may be heat or heating systems, which tend to overdry the air inside your home or office. This in turn dries out our upper respiratory passages, leaving them more vulnerable to viruses. Mucus serves to keep the germs constantly moving out of the nose, and when the flow slows or dries up, germs are more likely to linger and cause infection.

CAN THE FLU BE SHOT DOWN?

Just before flu season, toward the end of fall, people line up at company clinics or doctors' offices to get their flu shots in the hope of fighting off the bug before it can land. But is a flu shot a wise investment? If you're young and healthy, probably not. But if you belong to what physicians term the "high-risk" group—those who could develop serious problems if they get the flu—a flu shot is a wise move. This high-risk group includes people over 65, as well as those with chronic lung diseases, such as asthma or emphysema; heart disease; kidney disease; diabetes or severe anemia. These vaccinations are only a preventive measure and won't do a thing if you have already gotten the flu. For others, the younger and healthier folks, simply building up natural immunity will be the best defense against the flu.

VITAMINS THAT SWAT THE BUG

Nature has given us some natural weapons to zap colds and flu or even ward them off. Vitamin C is the winner in this department.

Terence Anderson, M.D., Ph.D., a Canadian doctor who specializes in

Sweating It Out

What do lying in bed with the flu and taking a dance class have in common? Something called endogenous pyrogen (EP), that's what. It's your body's own firestarter, and if the scientists are right, it's EP that makes your brow damp whether you're fighting off the latest loathsome bug or working out to "Saturday Night Fever." Moreover, doctors believe that EP plays an important role in fighting illness.

Does this mean, as some hasty observers have suggested, that you should jump into your gym shorts when you feel a cold coming on?

Such advice is "very dangerous," according to Joseph Cannon, Ph.D., the chief discoverer of the exercise/EP tie-in, who points out that there are hundreds of thousands of different diseases and that exercise might affect each differently. Exercise might actually spread a virus in its early stages by increasing blood flow, adds another doctor. (Massage or sauna might be hazardous in the early stages of an illness for the same reason.) And, warns Jeffrey Jahre, M.D., chief of the infectious disease section at St. Luke's Hospital, Bethlehem, Pennsylvania, exercise-induced fatigue can interfere with your body's defenses against disease.

But can regular exercise help you avoid colds and flu in the first place, as many people who work out believe? According to at least one study, the answer is yes. After 4 months on a schedule of 1½-hour workouts 3 times a week, a group of adults showed increased production of infection-fighting cells when compared with nonexercising groups. And the count was even higher for a group that took vitamin C and E in addition to working out.

vitamin C research, found that those who took large doses of the vitamin during the early days of a cold suffered a lot less from cold miseries

(continued on page 46)

Some Uncommon Cold Care Tips

There may be no cure for the common cold but that doesn't mean you have to hoist the white flag when cold germs and viruses invade the locale. Here are a few tips—and a few no-no's—that will help you prevent colds or minimize their blow.

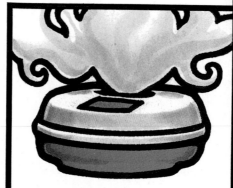

DO humidify your house, preferably at a 30 to 40 percent humidity level.

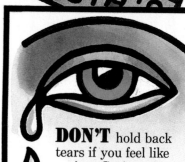

DO grow a beard, The hairs act as a filter against the cold virus. One doctor found that 70 percent of his patients with beards or mustaches weathered the flu season without a sniffle.

DON'T automatically use over-the-counter remedies and cough syrups. They often won't help you feel much better and can worsen symptoms. Antihistamines, which are contained in almost all over-the-counter remedies, can cause drowsiness and nausea, alter blood pressure in hypertensive people and thicken mucus in respiratory passages, worsening a cold. Many cough syrups contain alcohol, which dehydrates the body and lowers resistance.

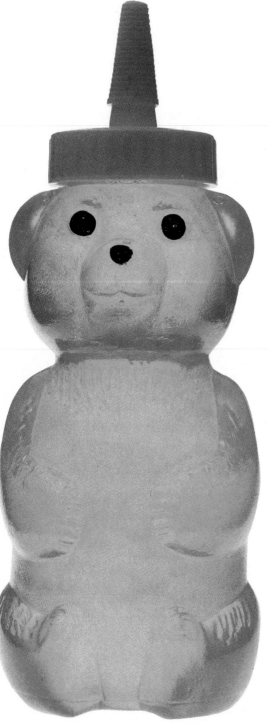

DO add some honey to your lemon tea, or gargle with honey and vinegar in hot water to relieve congestion, aches and cough.

DON'T hold back tears if you feel like crying. Crying provides an outlet for stress and thus helps keep up our body's defenses.

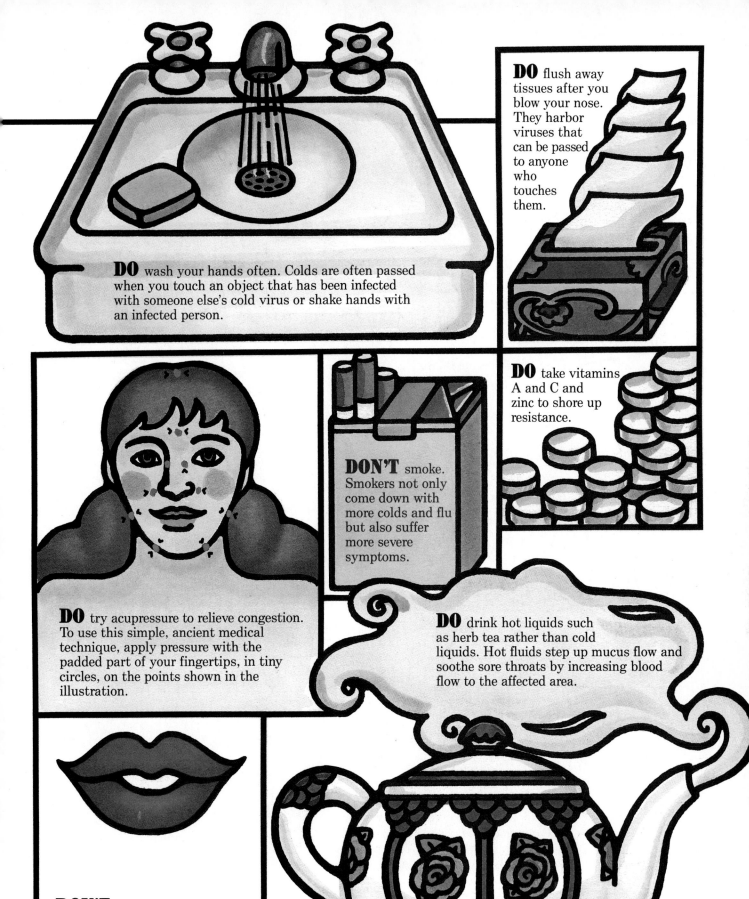

DO wash your hands often. Colds are often passed when you touch an object that has been infected with someone else's cold virus or shake hands with an infected person.

DO flush away tissues after you blow your nose. They harbor viruses that can be passed to anyone who touches them.

DO take vitamins A and C and zinc to shore up resistance.

DON'T smoke. Smokers not only come down with more colds and flu but also suffer more severe symptoms.

DO try acupressure to relieve congestion. To use this simple, ancient medical technique, apply pressure with the padded part of your fingertips, in tiny circles, on the points shown in the illustration.

DO drink hot liquids such as herb tea rather than cold liquids. Hot fluids step up mucus flow and soothe sore throats by increasing blood flow to the affected area.

DON'T kiss anyone during the early period of a cold or flu. The newer the infection, the more potent the virus.

and had about one-third fewer sick days. In his study, patients normally took just one 500-milligram tablet a week but tried 1,500 milligrams on the first day of a cold and 1,000 milligrams on days two through five.

Other researchers are finding that vitamin C bolsters the immune system—our squad of antibodies, proteins and special cells that fight viruses and bacteria. Richard Panush, M.D., chief of immunology at the University of Florida College of Medicine in Gainesville, first conducted studies of vitamin C's effects in a test tube and found it boosted a number of immune responses. Then, in a study of volunteers, Dr. Panush gave vitamin C to half of his subjects and a placebo to the remainder. Doctors measured immunity by analyzing the volunteers' blood samples for the presence of lymphocytes, germ-fighting cells. They found those who had taken vitamin C had enhanced immunity.

Many nutrition-oriented doctors believe that the Recommended Dietary Allowance of vitamin C—60 milligrams daily—is too low to truly brace our immunity, and say that supplementing your C intake is probably a wise move.

Vitamin A is another immune system booster that battles colds and flu. It especially aids the workings of the mucous membranes. Researchers in Thailand discovered that animals deficient in vitamin A had fewer germ-battling antibodies in their mucous membrane secretions. And vitamin A not only thins the mucus but also spurs the development of healthy mucus-producing cells. The constant movement of mucus through the respiratory tract keeps germs from settling there.

"TAKE TWO ZINCS . . ."

Another remedy from nature's pharmacy may come as a surprise: zinc. In one study, William W. Halcomb, D.O., and researchers George Eby and Donald Davis found that cold sufferers treated with zinc sliced the duration of colds by seven days. The study was begun after a child in their care refused to swallow a 50-milligram zinc gluconate tablet and instead let it dissolve slowly in her mouth. Her cold symptoms disappeared in a matter of hours. Dr. Halcomb then conducted a test on 65 patients who had had cold symptoms for three days or less. Thirty-seven patients were given dosages of two 23-milligram zinc tablets to start and one every

The Cold and Flu Sufferer's

MENU

Since colds and flu are caused by viruses, nothing we buy at the drugstore will effect a cure. But you can help your healing along simply by eating right.

Fever is dehydrating, so put plenty of liquids on your menu. Fruit juices help replenish blood sugar levels and the electrolytes (potassium, sodium and magnesium) lost through sweat. Hot liquids can do wonders to clear congestion. Researchers who compared the effects of hot chicken soup to plain water found that the soup increased the speed of mucus flow from the nose by 33 percent.

Another form of heat works well, too—spices. Hot, spicy foods stimulate blood flow, bringing a flood of antibodies to your sore throat. They also thin mucus and clear it out. Add garlic, horseradish, cayenne pepper and hot chilis to your recipes. Or try a gargle of 1 teaspoon of Tabasco sauce in a glass of warm water.

Steep a teaspoon of mullein, anise, horehound, hyssop or sage in boiling water and flavor with a dash of citrus juice to help clear congestion.

You should probably drink as many fluids as you can stand, but go easy on food. Cut down on heavy fats and proteins.

Finally, forget that hot toddy. Alcohol can actually lower your immunity, deplete your body of vitamins and dehydrate you even more.

two waking hours for a week; 28 other patients received a placebo. The researchers found that the 37 zinc-treated patients kept their colds an average of 4 days, compared with 11 days for the others. Dr. Halcomb theorizes that the mineral inhibits viral replication and bolsters the body's immunity. This treatment involves a lot of zinc and ought not to be continued for long periods or undertaken without a doctor's supervision.

THE HEALING FIRE

Fever, one of the first symptoms of colds and flu, may be one of the best indicators that the body is fighting the infection, since it indicates that our bodies are producing endogenous pyrogen (EP), a substance that triggers certain proteins to battle infection.

Fever is a natural response and one you need not necessarily rush to treat with drugs, says Alan K. Done, M.D. Dr. Done, who is president of the Association of Consulting Toxicologists, explains that too often, parents pressure physicians to treat their children for a fever even though fever can help monitor the intensity of an illness. Besides, infectious fevers rarely get out of control.

A SORE SIGN OF TROUBLE

When you have a runny nose, you usually know instantly that you've caught a cold. But a sore throat isn't such an easy signal for us to read. It could be simply due to overusing your voice or breathing in the winter air, which acts like a desert wind on the throat. Or it might indicate a more serious infection, like the flu, especially if it's accompanied by a fever above 101° or a red rash at the back of the throat. Most sore throats are caused by viruses, though some, like "strep" throat, are caused by bacteria.

An acute sore throat should disappear within a few days to a couple of weeks, but if it lasts

When a Tickle Means Trouble

Coughing may seem like a nagging inconvenience, but it's often productive: It helps to raise phlegm and clear the respiratory tract. Certain signs indicate more serious problems, however. It's time to see a doctor when:
- your cough has lingered more than 10 days.
- it's accompanied by fever that rises above 102° or lasts longer than 3 days.
- your cough seems to go away, but comes back shortly afterward.
- you cough up blood.
- your cough is painful or interferes with normal activities.
- you become short of breath.
- you cough up large amounts of mucus for more than 3 days.

longer, you'd better consult your doctor.

In the meantime, there's plenty you can do to relieve the tickling and scratching, pain or hoarseness. One good remedy is a tea or gargle of herbs or spices. Try 10 to 20 drops of Tabasco sauce in a glass of water, or use lots of horseradish, chili or mustard in your food. They increase the blood flow to your throbbing throat. Hot ginger milk is another comfort for the scratchy throat that accompanies sinus congestion. Heat, but don't boil, a cup or so of milk in a pan. Add two or three slices of fresh ginger to the milk, or if you don't have any fresh ginger root available, use ¾ to 1 teaspoon of ground ginger. Sucking on lemon, horehound or menthol lozenges can also soothe throat pain.

Many people feel they're not really battling a sore throat or similar complication until they've got a prescription for antibiotics in hand. They're probably choosing the wrong weapon, according to James Fries, M.D., and Donald Vickery, M.D. These doctors note that antibiotics are often used needlessly to treat sore throats, since the majority are due to viruses, and antibiotics combat bacterial infections. A throat culture is probably the best way to find out whether antibiotics are necessary. You can take a throat culture at home if you ask your doctor for a culture kit and a lesson.

Sexually Transmitted Diseases

Looking in the mirror, Donna felt more dread than excitement about her upcoming business trip to Dallas. Normally, she would have been as excited as a child ripping open a gift box at the thought of visiting a city where she had never been, sampling great restaurants and meeting interesting new clients of her advertising firm. But this time was different.

Donna gazed at the small, blistery bumps at the corners of her mouth, which had split open and felt sore. "How can I face my clients like this?" she muttered. "Why me?"

Donna is hardly alone. An estimated 500,000 persons each year come down with the same infection, sometimes accompanied by a fever and swollen gums.

The infection, known as herpes simplex virus Type I (HSV-I), oral herpes, fever blisters or cold sores, is just one of the illnesses that fall under the classification of "sexually transmitted diseases" (STDs). These medical problems, long known as venereal diseases, are now called sexually transmitted diseases, partly in an attempt to get away from the long-time stigma of the VD label, which prevented too many people from seeking treatment.

While the risks of certain STDs are potentially very serious—some may cause infertility or even cancer of the cervix if unheeded—most people's fears are exaggerated. Stories that focus on incurability have often alarmed more than informed. While STDs are prevalent, increased awareness of preventive measures, better diagnostic tests, new treatments and the trend to self-help are easing their impact.

HERPES: REASSURING NEWS

Oral herpes is a case in point. Often, like genital herpes, it is painted as incurable, and in the strict sense, it is. However, more than half of those who come down with oral herpes will never suffer a second infection, and only 5 to 10 percent of those with oral herpes will be bothered by repeated episodes throughout life.

Oral herpes is most often spread by mouth-to-mouth contact, but it can affect the genital area if oral-genital contact is made when one partner has an active cold sore. Since the virus is so contagious, a child can catch it even from a quick kiss from a relative who has cold sores, and HSV-I often occurs first in children under five years of age.

The initial infection is a little different from subsequent ones. Tiny ulcers can develop on the inside of the mouth and on the tongue, and may be so uncomfortable that they interfere with eating or drinking. These ulcers usually appear three to five days after the virus has been passed. Recurrent episodes are usually not as extensive as the initial outbreaks, although to the

"Can You Catch It from a Toilet Seat?"

Should you worry about catching herpes from public toilets? No, you shouldn't. That's the resounding answer from the medical profession. "The possibility of catching herpes this way is remote," says Neil H. Brooks, M.D., a Connecticut physician and past president of the Connecticut Academy of Family Physicians.

But what of research that revealed that herpes virus can live for hours on a dry toilet seat and up to days on such surfaces as cotton fabric? Doctors explain that unless your skin is broken, the herpes virus can enter your body only through mucous membranes such as the ones in your genital area, in your mouth or around your eyes. And mucous membranes do not come in contact with the toilet seat.

Despite the millions of cases of herpes in this country, there has not been a single confirmed case of the nonsexual transmission of the genital form of the disease. "One of my patients *said* he got it from a toilet seat," says Dr. Brooks, "but I know where he *really* got it."

sufferer they may still seem like a real eyesore.

While many people may think they can diagnose HSV-I by sight alone, the sores may resemble canker sores or impetigo, so the only sure way to know what they are is through a culture.

Knowing what triggers cold sores can help reduce recurrences. Overexposure to the sun's ultraviolet rays is the number one culprit in reactivating the virus, so if you are prone to oral herpes, one of your best investments may be a sunscreen with a sun protection factor of 15.

Other factors that can spur recurrences include any irritation of the mouth, lowered resistance from another infection such as the flu or a cold, or even emotional stress.

NUTRIENTS AS HEALERS

Nutrition may also play an important role in building resistance to herpes. Robert Peshek, D.D.S., who practices dentistry in Riverside, California, theorizes that cold sores reactivate when the body fails to absorb enough calcium. He advises his patients to take several nutrients to improve calcium absorption and stem other problems that contribute to cold sores. These nutrients include calcium fortified with magnesium (as in dolomite); essential fatty acids, which counter the effects of sun overexposure; acidophilus, the beneficial bacteria that helps maintain intestinal flora; and vitamin B complex, which tends to be low in herpes sufferers.

Dr. Peshek also warns those who are prone to fever blisters to avoid acidic foods, such as citrus fruits and juices, and high-fat foods, both of which inhibit calcium absorption. "I've treated several hundred patients this way, with a high percentage of success," he says.

At Hadassah University Hospital in Jerusalem, Israel, patients who had outbreaks of cold sores for

less than 48 hours were treated with a solution containing 4 percent zinc sulfate in water. (You can ask a pharmacist to make this mixture for you.) The solution was applied to the blisters four times daily for four days.

Every patient found that the pain, tingling and burning ceased within the first 24 hours of treatment. The sores crusted within one to three days, with no adverse effects reported Previously the blisters of the oral herpes patients had taken between four and ten days to crust over, the researchers noted.

At the health clinics of two companies in Liverpool, England, doctors gave their patients vitamin E capsules with instructions to prick the capsules with a pin and apply the liquid contents to the HSV-I lesions every 4 hours. The results were "striking"—the lesions disappeared quickly and the pain went away. The doctors later treated at least 50 patients successfully with the vitamin.

HERPES II CONTROL

Some 20 million Americans have contracted genital herpes, or herpes simplex virus Type II (HSV-II), and there are an estimated 300,000 new cases each year. Happily, less than 10 percent will be chronic sufferers.

Usually, HSV-II strikes below the waist and is passed through intimate contact with an infected person. In men, the lesions normally appear on and around the genitals, and even the buttocks and thighs. In women, the blisters can affect the external genital area as well as the vagina and cervix.

The first herpes attack feels a lot like the flu, with fever, aching muscles and swollen glands in the groin. Blisters soon pop out, usually accompanied by itching and burning. The first attack can take as long as two to three weeks to run its course. Should you contract these symp-

(continued on page 52)

Avoiding Arginine: The Antiherpes Diet

You probably don't think too often about the arginine content of the foods you eat, but if you suffer recurrent herpes attacks, you may want to start. This amino acid has been found to favor growth and reproduction of the herpes virus. Below are some common foods and ingredients high in arginine:
- Almonds
- Barley
- Bran
- Brussels sprouts
- Cashews
- Chocolate
- Coconut
- Corn
- Corn flakes
- Corn germ
- Cottonseed oil
- Gluten
- Macaroni
- Oats
- Peanuts
- Wheat germ

A Guide to Diagnosis, Self-Care and Medical Treatment

Infection	What It Is	Symptoms	Your Course of Action
Hemophilus vaginalis (HV)	A common form of vaginitis, or bacterial infection of the vagina.	Red, itchy vulva. Light discharge that looks and feels like flour paste (gray-white and sticky), and has a strong fishy odor. Painful urination and intercourse.	Salt-water bath before bed for 3 nights (½ cup salt in warm water). See a medical professional if symptoms persist.
Nongonococcal urethritis (NGU/NSU)	Any bacterial infection of the male reproductive tract other than gonorrhea.	Pain or burning on urination. Pus discharge.	Nondrug treatment involves cleansing out bacteria by drinking 10 glasses of water a day for 2 weeks. Eliminate coffee, alcohol.
Cystitis	Bacterial infection that can inflame the bladder and kidneys.	Uncomfortable and almost continual need to urinate. Burning on urination and sometimes blood in urine. Low abdominal pain, backache. Pain with intercourse.	Drink lots of water, at least 8 glasses a day. Cranberry juice is good substitute because acid in it inhibits bacterial growth. Avoid coffee and tea.
Chlamydia	Actually a series of related infections caused by intermediate organism *Chlamydia trachomatis.* Highly contagious.	Slight discharge. Painful intercourse; bleeding after intercourse. Burning on urination. Fever, chills, vomiting. Abdominal, back, leg, pelvic pain. No symptoms appear in early stages in 75% of cases.	See a medical professional immediately.
Herpes simplex virus Type II (HSV-II)	Virus commonly associated with lesions on genitals, and in women, in the cervix.	Clusters of small, painful or itchy blisters on genitals, buttocks or thighs, usually accompanied by local swelling. Fever, aching muscles and swollen glands in groin. Burning on urination. Recurrent infections may diminish in severity. Recurrences often start with itching, tingling, aching or burning at site of eventual outbreak.	Keep lesion clean and dry. Apply alcohol, peroxide or witch hazel directly to sore with cotton swab. Topical anesthetics like lidocaine may ease pain. Ice packs help swelling and discomfort. Warm baths with Epsom salts or baking soda can be soothing. Urination in a bathtub filled with water may help if otherwise painful. Supplement diet with lysine. See a medical professional before blisters break.
Candidiasis (Monilia)	Commonly known as "yeast infection," this is caused by a fungus growing in the vagina.	Red, itchy vulva. Cheesy-looking, yeasty-smelling discharge. Burning on urination. Painful intercourse. Bright red vagina with white patches on walls and cervix.	Insert boric acid powder packed in size 0 (600 mg.) gelatin capsules into vagina, 1 per night for 2 weeks. Salt-water bath before bed for 5 nights. Local application of yogurt. Low-sugar, yeast-free diet. Supplement diet with acidophilus. See a medical professional if symptoms persist after 1 week.
Trichomoniasis (Trich)	External infection of the female reproductive tract caused by protozoan organism *Trichomonas vaginalis.* A common form of vaginitis.	Vagina and vulva look wet and inflamed. Discharge that may be heavy, itchy, foamy, irritating, bad-smelling and gray-green in color. Lower abdominal pain. Painful intercourse. Tendency to worsen after menstruation. Frequent urination.	Salt-water bath before bed for 3 nights. See a medical professional if symptoms persist after several days.
Pelvic inflammatory disease (PID)	Serious infection that is often misdiagnosed; usually caused by either chlamydial or gonorrheal infection. Risk also heightened by use of IUD.	Earliest symptoms often go undetected. Fever, chills, lower abdominal pain, vaginal discharge (bloody or puslike), pelvic tenderness. Painful intercourse, bleeding after intercourse. Nausea, vomiting. Painful urination.	See a medical professional immediately.

☐ Bacteria	☐ Intermediate Organism	☐ Virus
☐ Protozoa	☐ Various Causes	☐ Fungus

Medical Diagnosis and Treatment	Important Facts
Diagnosis: Wet-mount smear; immediate results. "Whiff test": exposure of vaginal secretions to drop of 10% KOH solution yields characteristic fishy smell. Immediate but not definitive results. **Treatment:** Orally administered antibiotics, like ampicillin. Use of sulfa vaginal cream, Keflex, Flagyl.	Not serious but very annoying. Highly contagious. Responsible for most infections previously labeled nonspecific vaginitis.
Diagnosis: Distinguished from gonorrhea by microscopic examination of pus discharge. **Treatment:** Tetracycline.	Usually associated with fatigue, stress and poor diet. If taking tetracycline, avoid milk products and antacids.
Diagnosis: Laboratory analysis of urine sample to identify bacterial agent. **Treatment:** Antibiotics.	Annoying and inconvenient, but not a threat to general health. If untreated, infection can spread to kidneys.
Diagnosis: Specialized culture usually available only in well-equipped VD clinics or hospitals. Often made by process of elimination. **Treatment:** Orally administered antibiotics like tetracycline, sulfonamide, erythromycin.	Highly contagious. Can lead to pelvic inflammatory disease. Infected newborns can develop serious eye infections and pneumonia.
Diagnosis: Culture grown from tissue sample scraped from base of open blister (only definitive measure). Blood test. Frequently misdiagnosed. **Treatment:** New antivirals (acyclovir, adenine arabinoside) seem topically effective in primary attacks and only when used early in course of infection. Major drawbacks to these in present form (cream, ointment) is that they keep lesion moist. However, a 5-day course of acyclovir treatment may prevent new lesion formation and shorten healing time in recurrent episodes.	More than half of sufferers will never have second attack. Recurrence is related to general health—emotional, physical and strength of body's resistance. Creams containing cortisone should be avoided; they slow healing and may cause spread of virus. Women should be monitored carefully during pregnancy; virus can seriously affect infant infected by active lesion during birth.
Diagnosis: Wet-mount smear; immediate results. **Treatment:** Antifungal creams and suppositories like nystatin, miconazole, clotrimazole. Gentian violet.	Can damage vaginal walls, making them more susceptible to invasion by other bacteria. Newborns infected through vaginal delivery can get oral infection, which interferes with nursing.
Diagnosis: Culture; results in 5 days. Wet-mount smear; immediate results. (Only definitive for positive results.) Pap smear. **Treatment:** Vagisec, Flagyl.	Can cause changes in cervical cells which may increase chances of more serious cervical disease later on. Flagyl is only sure cure. New research indicates one large dose as effective as 7-day treatment and has fewer side effects.
Diagnosis: Gram stain. Culture. **Treatment:** Antibiotics like tetracycline, penicillin, ampicillin. Flagyl. Occasionally hospitalization is required.	Serious health problem. May be caused by bacterial or intermediate organisms that have migrated to the pelvic cavity. Misdiagnosed in more than one-third of all cases. Can cause salpingitis (infection of fallopian tube), which may promote sterility or tubal pregnancy. Also responsible for endometriosis, cysts, abscesses.

NOTE: Check with your practitioner about drug side effects and interactions. Pregnant women should be cautious of all oral medications and avoid Flagyl, podophyllin, some antifungal agents and some antibiotics, especially tetracycline. Nursing mothers should avoid Flagyl.

toms, you should see a doctor immediately, since the virus can be identified with certainty only through a culture or blood test. The physician can also prescribe an antiviral drug called acyclovir, which has prevented recurrences in some patients when used to treat their initial herpes attack.

Thankfully, as with oral herpes, subsequent attacks of genital herpes are usually much less severe than the first one as the body develops an immunity to the virus. A recurrence is usually signaled in advance by the "prodrome," a set of symptoms that includes tingling, itching or burning in the perineal or genital area; twitches, pain or tenderness of the groin and general weakness, like the onset of flu. The prodrome is important not only because it signals that herpes is about to recur but because it marks the beginning of the infection's contagion. (The contagious period ends when the blisters have dried and healed.) The prodrome usually occurs several hours or even days before the first sores erupt. Recurrences end more quickly than the first attack and run their course in about 5 to 10 days.

Serious complications of genital herpes are rare, but pregnant women must be especially cautious. A newborn can become infected with

the herpes virus during vaginal delivery if the mother has active lesions. If you are pregnant and suspect you have HSV-II, be certain to tell your doctor about the disease.

Another potential risk of both HSV-I and HSV-II is an eye infection transmitted when you touch an open herpes lesion and then rub your eyes. In rare cases, this infection can spread to the deeper layers of the cornea and cause blindness. So, if you contract herpes, wash your hands thoroughly before touching your eyes during the contagious period.

A statistical link has also been established between cancer of the cervix and genital herpes, although researchers have not found that herpes *causes* cervical cancer. If you contract herpes, it's a good idea to follow up with a Pap smear every 6 to 12 months.

LYSINE'S ROLE

Some people may actually be eating their way into recurrent herpes episodes when they choose foods containing a high amount of arginine, one of the amino acids. Scientists have found that arginine supports the growth and reproduction of the herpes virus. On the other hand, lysine, a second amino acid, has been found to inhibit the growth of the virus by lessening the amount of arginine the body absorbs during digestion.

Jonathan Wright, M.D., of Kent, Washington, who specializes in nutritional treatment, explains that the ratio of arginine to lysine in foods is critical. If a food has a high arginine-to-lysine ratio, it could set off herpes, while foods that have a higher lysine-to-arginine ratio could help cut herpes episodes short. Meat, potatoes, milk and brewer's yeast contain a large portion of lysine.

The results of experiments using lysine dietary supplements have been mixed. Various researchers have reported that dosages of from 500 to 1,000 milligrams a day help lessen pain and heal the lesions faster. But some studies that used

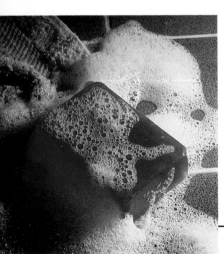

Watching the Soaps

If you're prone to urinary problems, you may have to look no further for the cause than the bar of soap in your bathroom. Several years ago, a doctor in Sweden, U. Ravnskov, studied 31 women who had recurrent urinary tract infections or dysuria (painful urination). He found that 27 of the women washed their genital area with soap 1 to 3 times a day. On the doctor's advice 22 of the women stopped using soap, washing only with water. Of the 22, 17 found the painful urination disappeared within 1 to 8 weeks, and never recurred. Dr. Ravnskov believes that overzealous use of soap is an even bigger culprit than bacteria in urinary tract infections.

control groups given placebos were less than promising. In one study of 21 patients with recurring herpes episodes, some subjects were given dosages of 400 milligrams of lysine three times a day, while others were given placebos. John DiGiovanna, M.D., and Harvey Blank, M.D., reported no beneficial effects in the lysine users.

Despite the absence of conclusive data, herpes sufferers might want to limit arginine in their diet, and more lysine couldn't hurt.

CHLAMYDIA: A NEW THREAT

Talk of sexually transmitted diseases usually centers on gonorrhea, syphillis and herpes. But another highly contagious infection has become epidemic: chlamydia (pronounced *kluh-MID-ia*). This type of STD now occurs between five and ten times as frequently as gonorrhea in women, and three times as often in men. Worse, it can often be misdiagnosed.

Chlamydia is caused by an intermediate organism (neither virus nor bacteria) that invades the mucus-producing cells that line the genital tract. The infection is as subtle as it is slow. Typically, the incubation period can last three weeks. Eventually, women will notice a slight discharge, pain during coitus and, later, lower abdominal pain and a fever. In men, the first signs of chlamydia are pain while urinating and a discharge from the urethra. When symptoms appear, it's important to seek medical attention immediately to control the infection.

The organism can pass through the reproductive tract of women, from the cervix to the uterine lining and to the fallopian tubes, if unchecked. There it can prompt pelvic inflammatory disease (PID), scarring the tubes and even resulting in infertility. Male sufferers of chlamydia have similar worries if the disease spreads. The infection can go from the urethra to the testicles, where it can prompt painful swelling and inflammation known as epididymitis and may result in sterility. Also,

more than half of what doctors used to call nonspecific urethritis (NSU), or nongonococcal urethritis (NGU), in men is believed to be caused by the chlamydial organism.

Once chlamydia is diagnosed, it can be readily treated with antibiotics. Be sure to follow your physician's prescription to the letter, even if your symptoms disappear, since the organism often resists treatment and requires a full course of antibiotics to squelch it.

THE TERMS OF ENDEARMENT

Although any intimate contact puts you at risk for sexually transmitted diseases, "women who have multiple sex partners are at highest risk for gynecological infections out of sheer probability from increased exposure," says Mary-Ann Shafer, M.D., associate director of the adolescent medicine unit, department of pediatrics, University of California at San Francisco. The same holds true for men, of course.

Your method of contraception can also have an impact on your susceptibility. Condoms, for instance, are considered the single most important barrier against sexually transmitted diseases and gynecological infections. They work in two ways: First, condoms prevent semen, a good culture medium for bacterial growth, from spilling into the vagina. Second, they act as a wall between the penis and the vagina, guarding against the transmission of organisms. The "bugs" they can stop include *Trichomonas, Hemophilus vaginalis* and *Chlamydia.*

Doctors are still debating whether the herpes virus can pass through the pores of a condom. "No one knows for sure whether condoms protect against herpes," says Dr. Shafer. "But until we know, use a condom between herpes attacks and abstain from intercourse during them."

Other Infections

John was very adept at hiding his sinking curve ball from opposing batters on other high school teams— and equally adept at hiding dirty socks from his mother. Whenever she gathered the laundry, she searched her son's duffle bag for dirty socks, to no avail. John was hiding his "lucky" socks inside his gym locker and wore them repeatedly before he finally handed them over to his mom. But one day John's careless hygiene caught up with him—he noticed a red, scaly rash between his toes. John had athlete's foot.

This fungal infection is very common during and after adolescence. The most prevalent (and persistent) fungal infection, athlete's foot is the bane of many who share a locker room or showers, since fungi thrive in warm, moist places.

In addition to the rash and itching, the skin between the toes usually cracks, causing pain and more severe itching. Preventive foot care can often fend off this troublesome problem (see "Private Health in Public Places").

GETTING RID OF IMPETIGO

Warm, moist conditions play a part in spreading impetigo. This highly contagious bacterial infection, which usually appears on the skin around the mouth and nose, is caused by the streptococcus or staphylococcus bacteria.

Impetigo usually starts as a small patch of tiny blisters or sores that feel tender, itchy or burning. Eventually, the blisters rupture and reveal moist, seeping skin underneath them. Slowly, the skin turns into a hardened crust that looks like brown sugar. The infection can spread at the edges to other areas. Although impetigo can appear quite sore and ugly, and be very persistent, it heals without scarring.

Mostly, the infection is spread through direct contact with the moist discharges from the lesions, but clothing or linens can also harbor the bacteria. Once you have impetigo, it's wise to seek medical attention, but there are some steps you can take to treat it at home, too. Clean the sores with water and an antibacterial soap, and wipe the affected area with alcohol. Remove the crusts by gently soaking the area with a saline (salt) solution, and follow this with an application of an antibiotic salve. Be sure to wash your hands thoroughly after soaking the sores. Also, wash your clothes and linens in hot water to keep the bacteria from spreading.

Doctors usually prescribe antibiotics like penicillin or erythromycin for impetigo. The infection should clear up within seven to ten days.

PINKEYE BLUES

Pinkeye, or conjunctivitis, is a highly contagious infection that strikes the conjunctiva, the membrane lining the eyelid. It's marked by a smarting, itching, gritty feeling, a pus discharge and pink streaks of inflammation running across the white of the eye. Children get it most often, but adults can come down with pinkeye as well.

Pinkeye strikes when the conjunctiva becomes inflamed from a viral or bacterial infection, smoke or particles of dust, foreign bodies in the eye, intense light, searing wind or allergies. When pinkeye is caused by an infection, it can also be spread readily through contaminated handkerchiefs, washcloths or other linens. The pus discharge is usually heavier in the bacterial infections than in allergic reactions.

Use warm water to flush your eyes thoroughly and wash away the discharge. If there is no itching or burning, apply warm wet compresses to the eyes for 15 minutes at a time, using this treatment three or four times a day. At its worst, pinkeye can make the eyelids stick together in the mornings, but warm compresses can open them again. If your pinkeye is caused by a bacterial infection, your doctor can prescribe antibiotic drops or ointment to apply after you have washed your eyes of the discharge.

Private Health in Public Places

Mary and Joan decided one day to relax in the hot tub at the new health spa downtown. The next day, both experienced lower abdominal pain and urinary tract infections. When health officials examined the hot tub, they found it had no working filter and had been chlorinated very little since it was built; it was therefore contaminated.

These women rudely discovered an unfortunate consequence of the fitness boom: locker rooms, saunas—any place where people sweat together—can be hotbeds of infection if they're not properly maintained. From athlete's foot to hot-tub dermatitis (a bothersome and itchy rash), such infections can make life temporarily miserable. Here are a few tips to help you protect yourself.

1 Locker rooms, steam rooms and showers are among the prime sites for athlete's foot fungus, which thrives in warm, moist places. To keep athlete's foot from taking hold, use rubber slippers in damp, tiled areas. Wear cotton or cotton and wool blend socks and dry your feet thoroughly before putting on shoes. Canvas sneakers or sandals are best for athlete's foot sufferers because they allow moisture to evaporate.

2 Powder your feet to keep them dry, using an over-the-counter foot powder with antifungal properties, says Mitchell Feingold, D.P.M. Don't use powders with a cornstarch base—they're a great medium for bacterial growth.

3 Neither borrow nor lend your towel and washcloth. They're very *personal* property, since they can act as vehicles for bacteria. Two threats they pose: conjunctivitis, or pinkeye, a common inflammation of the membrane lining the eyelids, and impetigo, a blistery, troublesome skin infection that looks like oral herpes.

4 The organism that prompts the itchy rash of hot-tub folliculitis can lurk in a sloppily maintained hot tub, especially when the water pH is too high. Health guidelines call for pH readings between 7.4 and 7.8. Chlorine levels are also critical. In public hot tubs and whirlpools the chlorine level should be from 4 to 6 parts per million (ppm), while a home hot tub should be kept at 2 to 3 ppm.

4

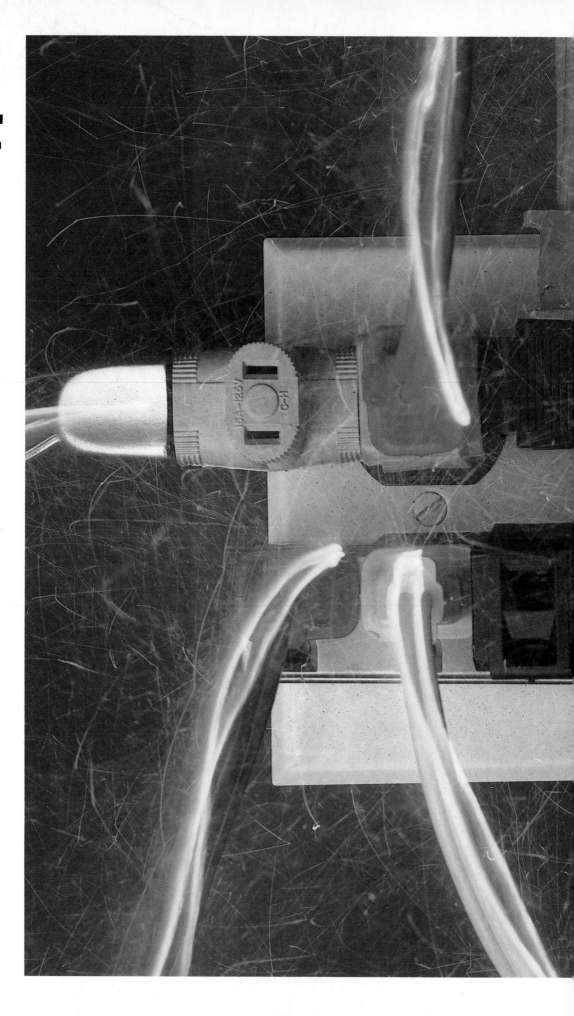

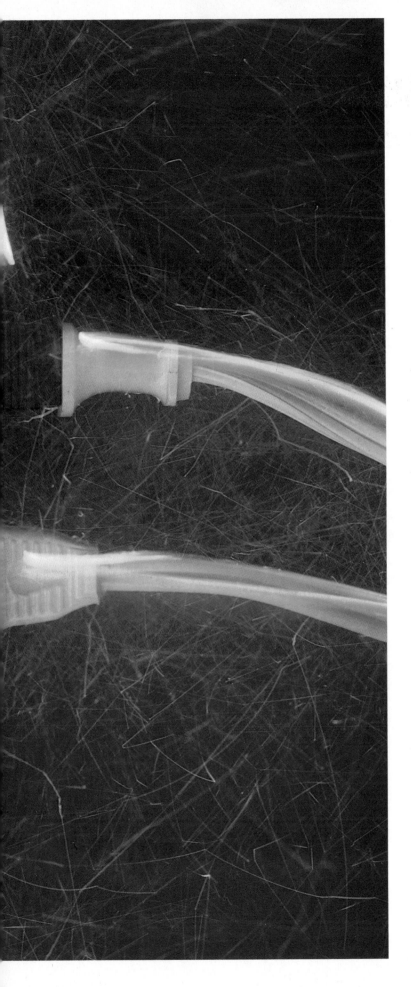

What to Do When You Overdo

Whether you've worked too hard or played too hard, you can still have a healthy morning after.

Y ou're concerned about good health and take pains to ensure you maintain it. So you'd be happy if you lived a life that didn't stray far from this pattern: frequent twilight strolls (but never to the ice cream parlor for chocolate brownie sundaes); afternoon touch football games where the winning team gets first dibs on the lemonade (no beer allowed); holiday get-togethers with the whole family gathered around small plates piled low with sensible servings of vegetables, brown rice and lean turkey (no roasts or gravy, thank you).

You would be happy, right?

Of course not. Everyone needs the thrill of splurging or acting recklessly once in a while. What would life be without occasional overindulgence on festive occasions? There would be less indigestion and fewer hangovers, but there would also be less fun. You shouldn't berate yourself for overdoing it once in a while. But you should quickly take care of the symptoms of overindulgence so you can get on with your healthy life. This chapter will show you how to do just that, with drug-free remedies.

Other types of overdoing it aren't so much fun. Sometimes we overextend ourselves not because we want to, but because we have to fulfill obligations to our job and to others. This type of overdoing it often results in fatigue, listlessness, boredom and general burnout—dangerous feelings that can lead you deep into the dumps. Often these feelings are diagnosed as purely psychological, but actually, there are many physical causes. You can stop burnout and fatigue before they begin to fester by taking positive action. The right diet helps. So does getting enough sleep and exercise. Read on for the best natural prescription to beat the symptoms of overdoing it.

Fighting Fatigue

You see them every day—people brimming with life. They exercise, put in long, creative hours at work, help their kids with their homework and still have enough energy to cook a three-course meal, clean up *and* read the latest best-seller or take in a movie. These happy, energetic people are the envy of the rest of us—normal people who, though generally fit and alert, suffer occasional bouts of fatigue that leave us behind in our work, irritable and wishing there were an easier way to get through the day.

Well, thankfully, there is. And we don't mean a visit to a doctor, only to hear that "it's all in your

A High-Energy Wake-Up for Slow Starters

You're familiar with the sensation: Your mind is awake, but your body is still asleep. You lie still in your bed, waiting until the last minute to crawl out from under the covers and get ready to face the day. Here's why: While you sleep, your circulation slows down, your body temperature drops and your muscles become stiff and cold from lack of movement. But you don't have to start your day feeling like a barely warm corpse. Rouse your body gently, and you'll start off your day with more pep than you knew you had. This routine will give you that needed jump on the day.

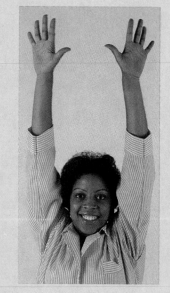

1 Before you get out of bed, raise your arms and slowly rotate your wrists. Open and close your hands a few times. Then lower your arms as you take a deep breath and push out your belly. Exhale slowly.

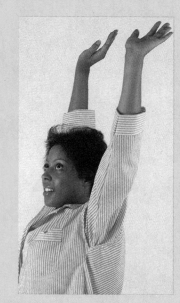

4 Raise your arms over your head and behind you as far as you can. Inhale deeply, expanding your belly. Lower your arms and exhale slowly. This deep breathing will really perk up your body.

5 Slowly roll out of bed and walk around your bedroom a few times. Your body temperature will immediately rise to meet the day, and your muscles will loosen.

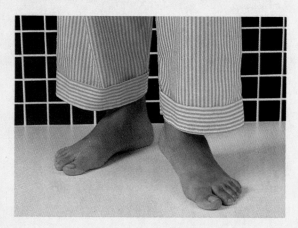

head," which in itself can be pretty tiring, or to get a prescription for a tranquilizer to make you less tense. You can eliminate most fatigue with simple, natural methods like eating high-energy foods, exercising regularly and getting enough sleep. (Of course, if you've got long-standing fatigue or you suddenly develop a case of severe tiredness, check it out with your doctor. It may mean a health problem too serious for self-care.)

LOWERING THE SHEEP COUNT

"Insomnia is a major cause of

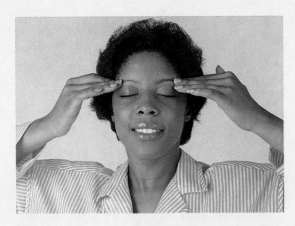

2 Press down along the line of your eyebrows with the tips of your fingers. Follow by rubbing your temples. Repeat this massage several times.

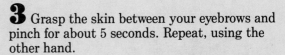

3 Grasp the skin between your eyebrows and pinch for about 5 seconds. Repeat, using the other hand.

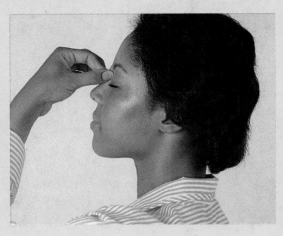

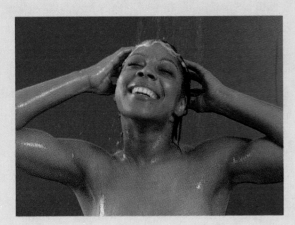

6 Take a warm shower. The heat and rhythmic pounding of the water will help you convince your body that it's time to wake up and get moving.

7 If you like to exercise in the morning, do it gently. Now that you've taken a shower, you'll feel more supple and enjoy the stretches more.

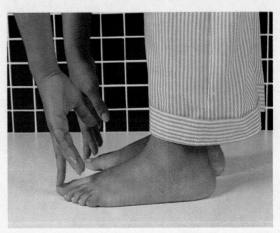

Nutrition to Spark Your Energy

Perhaps the most talked-about nutritional fatigue fighter is *iron*. This mineral helps the body manufacture hemoglobin, a protein in the blood responsible for delivering oxygen to every tissue and cell. Without iron, oxygen delivery slows, and the body doesn't get the energy it needs. Women need almost twice as much iron as men because of losses during menstruation, yet studies show that most women don't get enough; therefore, they should pay special attention to their iron intake. Good sources of iron include liver, lean ground beef, lima beans, soybeans and sunflower seeds.

Vitamin C helps with the absorption of iron, so be sure your diet includes plenty of C-rich fruits and vegetables, like strawberries, citrus fruits, cantaloupe, cabbage, peppers and broccoli. And vitamin C alone has been shown to raise the body's energy level. In one study, workers given 1,000 milligrams of vitamin C a day reported less fatigue and faster reaction times than before.

The B vitamins *folate* and B_{12} also work together to help form healthy red blood cells. Folate is found in brewer's yeast, cantaloupe and broccoli. For vitamin B_{12}, make sure you get enough poultry, fish, eggs, dairy products and meat.

Finally, make certain you are getting enough *magnesium*, a mineral that sparks dozens of crucial chemical reactions in the body. Mild magnesium deficiency has only one symptom: fatigue. Researchers studied 200 men and women who were tired during the day. After being given magnesium, all but 2 people reported that their tiredness had disappeared.

C Mg B Fe B12

fatigue," says Timothy Monk, Ph.D., assistant professor of psychology in the department of psychiatry at Cornell Medical College, White Plains, New York. Yet, as most insomniacs know, getting more sleep is easier said than done. At night your body may be dog-tired, but your mind is just dogged—a bloodhound that sniffs at the mental tracks of every worry, pressure and upset you experienced that day. And when you wake up in the morning (after a few hours of fitful sleep), you sometimes feel *more* tired than when you hit the sack—as if a sack's been hitting *you*. One way to beat insomnia-caused fatigue is to pay attention to your body's energy fluctuations, called circadian rhythms.

These natural rhythms work together like the musicians in an orchestra. When every musician follows the baton, each one comes in at the right time. But when there's no conductor, the beat becomes irregular. The various elements of your schedule—when you get up and go to bed, when you eat and exercise, how long you work—are the musicians that you orchestrate. And if you're troubled with insomnia, one musician you want to retire is daytime napping.

"You can get into a cycle of napping and then staying up late if you nap during the day," says Dr. Monk. Instead you should try—no matter how tired you feel—staying awake all day and then going to bed at the same time every night, even if you don't feel tired. The theory is that if you stick to this regular schedule, the energy rhythms of your body and mind will soon catch on that they're supposed to shut down at night and be active during the day. In short, you'll operate like clockwork.

EAT, DRINK AND BE TIRED

Some things people take into their bodies almost universally produce fatigue. Too much alcohol is one obvious example. Cigarettes also cause fatigue because smoking increases the body's need for oxygen at the same time it reduces the supply, tiring the body and interfering with sleep. Coffee, too, has deleterious effects. The letdown that comes as a caffeine high wears off can result in fatigue and lethargy, according to Sanford Bolton, Ph.D., of St. John's University in Queens, New York. Too much sugar can also cause fatigue by sending blood sugar levels (which help control energy) on a roller coaster ride.

Still, don't think that self-denial is the only way to beat fatigue. There are foods you can add to your diet that will help you pep up naturally. A team of researchers in Morristown, New Jersey, had 58 breakfast-skippers eat high-protein morning meals that included foods like fish, meat or cheese, flavored gelatins and brewer's yeast. They were also told to reduce their intake of sugar. The results: 49 of the 58 "reported obvious, in some instances dramatic, reductions in fatigue," because the added protein and the absence of sugar helped prevent fluctuations in blood sugar. Another way to keep blood sugar balanced is to eat six small meals a day instead of three large meals. This keeps the body supplied with a steady amount of blood sugar—making your day more like a cruise through the tunnel of love than a ride on a roller coaster.

THE AFTERNOON BLUES

Midafternoon fatigue is a common problem, judging by the rate at which office coffee pots empty around 3 P.M. There is a simple alternative to caffeine, however. Dr. Monk says, "If you want to stay alert in the afternoon, have a light lunch. Avoid bread, potatoes and other starchy foods." Try vegetables, cold lean meat or soup instead. If you eat a light lunch but still get the midafternoon blahs, try this simple perk-up exercise: 25 jumping jacks.

You may not have done this exercise since you were in junior high, but don't dismiss jumping jacks as child's play. Your minute of jumping will double your body's blood flow, mobilize the liver to release carbohydrates into the blood, giving you an energy boost, and raise your metabolism and oxygen intake by anywhere from 25 to 75 percent.

If that doesn't jack up your energy levels, nothing will.

While a short exercise break will give you a temporary boost,

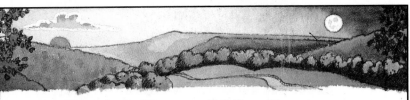

Timing Yourself for Energy

Do you find yourself saying you're a "night person," or trying to avoid morning meetings because you just can't think straight before noon?

According to management consultant Dorothy Tennov, Ph.D., everyone has high- and low-energy periods. The trick, she says, is taking advantage of the highs.

She suggests that you divide your energy state into 5 levels: level 1 for peak periods when you can apply yourself creatively to your work; level 2 for periods of slightly less energy; and so on down to level 5, where you just feel like watching television or daydreaming. Spend a week recording your levels on the hour, each hour you are awake.

Then analyze the results and schedule your most important, demanding work around energy levels 1 and 2. If you peak soon after you wake up, for instance, try completing your most difficult work—like a report for the boss or your tax return—early in the morning. "The rhythms are remarkably stable," says Dr. Tennov. "The increase in my productivity when I took full advantage of my high-energy periods was huge."

regular exercise will have beneficial long-term effects on your fatigue. Try running, walking, swimming or any other heart-building exercise for 30 minutes three or four times a week—you'll be impressed with the results. You'll probably lose weight and gain muscle tone, so you won't have as much body fat to drag around. Plus, your body will utilize glycogen—the fuel your muscles burn—and oxygen better. Exercise not only helps you use these fuels more efficiently, it also expands your fuel storage capacity—by up to twice as much. The bottom line: Exercise gives you more energy than if you just sat around resting, waiting for your fatigue to disappear.

Job Burnout

Sometimes it's hard to tell if your feelings of overwork, strain or on-the-job boredom are really symptoms of burnout. A California psychiatrist has developed a test to help you decide whether burnout is really what ails you.

Each symptom has been ranked with a number in the left-hand column marked "symptom points." For each symptom you experience, circle the symptom points, then rate its duration, intensity and frequency on the 1-3 scale indicated in each column. At the end, total your ratings and the symptom points you circled. Rate yourself according to the following scale:

0-20: No burnout potential
21-60: Possible burnout potential
61-100: Definite burnout potential
101 and over: Danger signal. See your doctor.

Your job is getting to be too much—too much boredom, repetition and frustration. It's as though you were hanging from a cliff, clutching a lifeline with all your strength, wishing you could climb. Instead you slip, first 5 feet, then 10. The oily rope allows no grip, and you slide to the bottom knot. You're at the end of your rope, and you see nothing below.

Welcome to job burnout. It's a common problem; an estimated one in three sick days is taken due to fatigue. But if you catch burnout in the early stages, you'll be able to pull yourself back to solid ground.

A survey conducted by *Psychology Today* magazine found that the most common methods people use to cope with job burnout are overeating, overdrinking, smoking too much and daydreaming. All of these, except daydreaming (in moderation), are negative reactions that will just increase your fatigue and despair.

The simplest, most effective initial step to take is to change your routine. "Take a break from your work," advises Stephan D. Schuster, Ph.D., a psychologist and management consultant in Los Angeles. "Meditate, take a walk and relax at lunch—or do whatever fits your personality. Type A people won't want to meditate, but they won't mind jogging or playing racquetball."

Indeed, the latter type of break may serve an additional purpose. Exercise helps beat the fatigue that is a common symptom of job burnout. A group of Exxon employees in New York were tested during a six-month exercise program. At the end of the period, they had an increased capacity for work, and most said they were less tired at the end of each workday. You can exercise by taking a daily walk, jogging several times a week or riding an exercise bicycle. Choose the workout that fits your personality and your level of fitness.

Your time away from work is as important to your well-being on the job as those hours you spend with your nose to the grindstone. "The

Are You Burned Out?

Symptoms	Symptom Points	How Long 1 weeks 2 months 3 years	How Often 1 occasionally 2 frequently 3 all the time	How Intense 1 mild 2 moderate 3 severe	Total Points
Energy level decreased	2				
Sleep decreased	2				
Sleep increased	1				
Head or back pain	1				
Intestinal problems	2				
Appetite increased or decreased	1				
Shortness of breath	1				
Colds and sinus problems	2				
Use of tranquilizers	5				
Use of alcohol	5				
Bored	3				
Obsessed	4				
Depressed	3				
Irritable	4				
Jealous	3				
Defensive	4				
Too critical of self and others	4				
Grand Total					

happiest executives get most of their satisfaction outside of the office," says Dr. Schuster. "Your job does not have be your major source of ego satisfaction." Try to get involved with community groups, volunteer work or hobbies that have nothing to do with your job. That way, you won't base the worth of your whole life on the satisfaction you get—or fail to get—from your job.

And remember, mild burnout is normal; that's why we have vacations. Take advantage of your weekends and vacations. If you have trouble breaking away from work, make reservations with an advance, nonrefundable deposit to make it harder to cancel at the last minute.

How to Handle a Workaholic Boss

Your boss spent his last vacation in California, but not at the beach. Instead, he toured the factories that make parts for your company's new line of appliances. He routinely puts in 12-hour days, and you've heard it said that he can't fall asleep at night if his secretary forgets to mark it on his pocket calendar.

He's a workaholic and assumes that you are, too. But you're not, and now he wants you to work on the quarterly report during your vacation. What can you do?

According to Michael L. Silverman, Ed.D., a specialist in on-the-job stress, it's up to you to tell the boss he's being unrealistic. Workaholics need to be reminded that not everyone equates leisure time with wasted time. Negotiate a solution before the problem gets out of hand. Tell your boss that long hours are okay occasionally but not all the time, and ask for direction in how to allocate your time. Asking for help is not a sign of weakness or incompetence; it's a strong way to initiate negotiations.

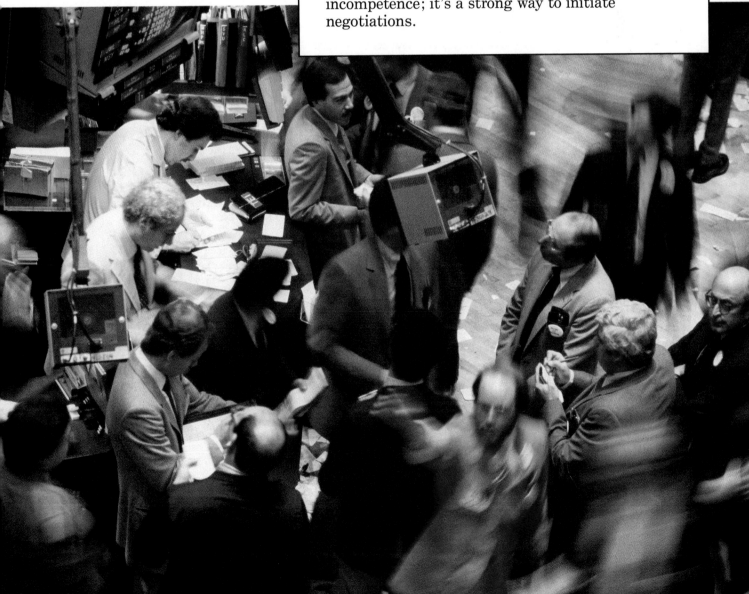

Eat, Drink and Still Be Merry

Better Ways to Spell Relief

The next time you suffer from indigestion, don't automatically reach for antacid tablets, which are often high in harmful sodium and aluminum. Here are some natural remedies that readers of *Prevention* magazine have found effective.

Papaya Enzyme Tablets. Available at most vitamin counters, they may help you digest food.

Parsley. A few sprigs of fresh parsley, or ¼ teaspoon dried parsley, taken with a glass of water, may relieve indigestion.

Olive Oil. Two tablespoons may help relieve stomach irritation.

Grapefruit Peel. Grate the outer skin down to the white layer, dry the grated bits and chew them slowly. This may help improve your digestion.

Celery. Chewing a stalk may help relieve heartburn.

Raw Potato. Take a piece of raw potato the size of your thumb, chew it well and swallow it. This may be good for a "sour" stomach.

Peppermint or Spearmint Tea. These herb teas have been used for gas and indigestion, but avoid peppermint if you have heartburn.

It doesn't take a physicist to prove that what goes up comes down, and neither does it take a physician to tell you that when you overeat, you pay the price; your stomach sends you the bill very quickly. Still, many of us are gluttons for punishment. We crave the experience of overindulging in food and drink so much that we repeatedly endure the consequences of our unrealistic appetites— anxiety, indigestion, tiredness.

"What these symptoms do is remind you not to overeat again, or at least avoid doing it in the near future," says David A. Levitsky, Ph.D., professor of nutrition and psychology at Cornell University. "Fortunately," he says, "the effects of occasional overeating are quite trivial." Trivial or not, however, bouts with gluttony usually end up leading to periods of discomfort.

So, what's the best way to spell relief? According to Dr. Levitsky, it's not in the dictionary—or the medicine chest. "The thing to do is make the most of the occasion. Sit back and experience the sensation of overeating. Take a nap if you feel tired," he says. In other words, don't berate yourself if you overeat—but don't make gluttony a habit, either.

Many people find relief with a brisk walk in the fresh air an hour or so after dinner. Others delight in hearing themselves groan. Whichever you choose, remember that your discomfort will go away in time. And try to eat lightly and exercise the next day to make up for your excess.

HOPE FOR HANGOVERS

Few examples of overdoing it follow the maxim, "you pay for your play," more strictly than overindulgence in spirits. The first few drinks may make you feel like you're floating on air, but if you have too many, you'll wake up thinking you fell head-first from your perch. Hangovers seem to be nature's way of telling you to take it easy.

Still, most people occasionally cast caution to the wind and awake after a night on the town nauseated, tired and headachy. The cause? There are several: toxins called congeners found in alcohol, dehydration, swollen arteries in the head and poor sleep. While the following treatments shouldn't be used as an excuse to get tipsy frequently, they will help you recover from a bout with the bottle.

The first is a preventive measure: Never drink on an empty stomach. Food, especially fat, will slow the absorption of the alcohol (some nightclubs in Japan serve squares of raisin butter just for this purpose). Second, limit your intake to one drink or glass of wine or beer an hour. This is the rate at which most people metabolize alcohol.

The final bit of preparation for an evening of drinking should be a healthy dose of vitamins. Many people recommend taking vitamins the morning after, but Warren M. Levin, M.D., of the World Health Medical Group in New York City, believes vitamins "should be taken at the time of error in judgment." That means take them before or while you drink.

Dr. Levin suggests that his patients fortify their system with vitamin C, B complex, zinc and magnesium. These supplements should help offset the vitamin and mineral leaching that takes place when you drink.

SWEAT YOUR BLUES AWAY

While the last thing on most people's minds after they've had one too many is a brisk walk or run around the neighborhood, exercise may be what's needed to save yourself from a morning after of moans and groans. Scientists at the University of Texas, in Austin,

Hung Over? Call a Cab

The medical study started with a party and ended with this sobering fact: Driving with a hangover can be as dangerous as driving when drunk.

Swedish researchers invited 22 paid volunteers to their lab for a little Friday night revelry fueled by appetizers, cocktails and dinner (accompanied by wine and beer, of course). The fun ended at midnight—the researchers wanted to induce hangovers, not major illness—and the soused subjects were put to bed in the lab. They awoke with hangovers to face a dizzying test: weaving a Volvo through a maze of pylons.

Though all were financially motivated (each bumped pylon cost them part of their pay), 19 of the subjects drove significantly worse with a hangover than they did normally—even though their blood alcohol levels had dropped to zero.

And, according to the researchers, the subjects drove poorly even when they reported "feeling fine." The lesson? Don't underestimate the lingering effects of alcohol.

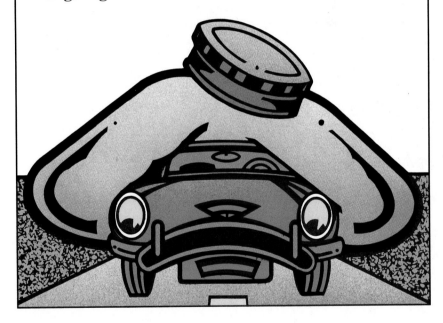

induced lab rats to drink intoxicating amounts of pure alcohol and later got them to run on treadmills. The result: Exercise accelerated the rate at which alcohol left the animals' bodies. "While this study was performed on rats, it's possible that it would have the same effect on humans," says researcher Carlton K. Erickson, Ph.D., professor of pharmacology at the university. The lesson for potential hangover sufferers is simple: Get out and get going to get over it.

Overexertion

The desire for a healthy heart, clear head and trim figure leads many people on an ill-fated quest for instant fitness. They push themselves too hard and wind up injured or too tired and discouraged to continue their exercise program.

But exercise needn't be a painful chore. In fact, says Michael D. Wolf, Ph.D., exercise scientist and author of *The Better Back Book,* "there is no logic to the old adage, 'no pain, no gain.' Pain means trouble."

The first step in preventing injury is to take it easy (this applies to moving furniture, chopping wood and other tasks, too). "You're trying to get fit for the rest of your life, right? Why go crazy trying to get in shape for this evening?" asks Dr. Wolf. "Why rush? Why jog in place at a stoplight when the light is red? Stop and stretch and rest for a few seconds instead. You'll still have a positive training effect, and you'll be less likely to injure yourself during the run."

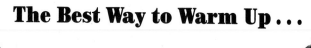

The Best Way to Warm Up . . .

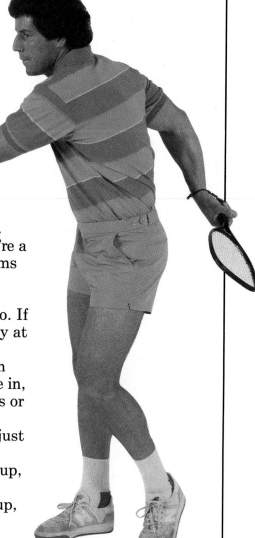

Warming up will make your workout more comfortable and less exhausting. When you put on your exercise clothes and rush immediately into your workout, you force your body to play catch-up: Your heart has to move from 1st to 4th gear so that your body gets enough oxygen, and your muscles have to quickly boost their temperature so they'll be flexible. This puts quite a strain on your system.

Instead, start out gradually. If you're a beginner, walk gently and move your arms and legs around to get the joints limber. Then ease into a slow jog, bike ride or whatever activity or sport you plan to do. If you're in good shape, just exercise slowly at first, without the added arm and leg movements, so that your body will warm up. No matter what kind of shape you're in, it's a good idea to warm up for 5 minutes or so if you're working out in the morning, because your muscles are cold and stiff just after you get up from bed.

Also, never stretch before warming up, because you'll risk injuring your cold muscles. If you feel stiff after warming up, feel free to stretch.

Bryant Stamford, Ph.D., director of exercise physiology at the University of Louisville, also says training too hard is a major factor in injuries, especially among recent converts to exercise. "You should always be conservative when you're training. Increase your workouts gradually, so you won't injure yourself."

It's also important to give your body a rest between exercise sessions. When you use your muscles during exercise, you deplete their energy stores and stress the tissue, so your muscles need time to rebuild themselves. Weight lifters often take a day off after each training day or work a different muscle group each day. And runners should run every other day or run a long distance one day and just a short distance the next.

Another good way to keep from overexerting yourself is to follow the whistle rule: Don't exercise to the point where you are breathing so heavily that you can't carry on a conversation, whistle or hum.

The whistle rule applies only while you are exercising, but overexertion will drag you down even off the court or track. You can tell if your training routine is chipping away at your overall health by monitoring your resting heart rate. First, get an accurate average measurement by checking your pulse in the morning while you are still in bed. Then keep a log of your heart rate on subsequent mornings. If you notice a sudden increase, you're probably overtraining. (Or you could be coming down with something.) Dr. Wolf lists several other signs of overtraining:

- General fatigue.
- Change in the quality and length (a lot more or a lot less) of sleep.

- Unusual weight loss, even though you've been eating the usual amount of food.
- Excessive, unusual thirst.

"If any of these symptoms occur, simply cut down on your training and see if they go away. Go for quality exercise, not quantity," says Dr. Wolf.

If you feel pain while working out, stop immediately. "Anytime you have a pain, your body is telling you something is wrong," says Dr. Stamford. This is especially true of joint pain. A "minor" joint injury can easily turn into a major problem, especially if you continue to exercise despite your injury.

Finally, be sure to rest until the injury has completely healed. Otherwise, you'll risk making a bad situation worse.

REST ASSURED

Don't think that a period of rest will offset all the gains you've made while exercising. Dr. Wolf cites many examples of athletes whose performances were actually helped by rest. "It's the new exercise tool for the 80s," he says. "One swimmer got sick seven weeks before a championship meet, and was forced to rest until the meet. People thought it would kill his performance, but he set three records. The rest actually helped him." Granted, says Dr. Wolf, "most people will lose their edge if they're out with an injury for two or three days. But even if you're out for a week, you won't have to start your training all over. After you're healed, resume exercising at a less strenuous rate than before the injury, just to play it safe. You'll soon be back to normal — without injury. A healing rest does much more good than harm."

...and Cool Down

Most people just want to stop and rest immediately after a race or workout, but there are very important reasons to cool down gradually, says Joel E. Dimsdale, M.D., of Harvard University. First, a cool-down period lets your body return blood from the extremities to the brain and heart, so you won't feel faint. Second, a cool-down period will prevent the release of too many hormones, called catecholamines, that can trigger irregular heartbeats, a real danger for people with heart disease. Dr. Dimsdale says the best way to avoid these problems is to walk at an easy pace for 5 minutes at the end of your workout, then lie on your back until you feel rested.

Eyestrain

Your eyes are your window on the world. When your vision is crisp and the leaves on the trees and the lines on a page are clear, everything makes more sense and you feel good. But when your vision is blurred, you have to strain to focus. You feel tired, overworked and headachy.

These feelings may simply be a natural response to a common problem: overwork. "The muscles in your eyes become fatigued after a long day," says Jerry Rapp, Ph.D., associate professor and chairman of biological sciences, State University of New York College of Optometry, in New York City. Whether the overuse is due to uncorrected vision problems, poor lighting or just too much work, your eyes grow weary. "Focusing—repeatedly shifting focus as the eyes glance from a close object to the far wall, from the road to the car radio—involves manipulating the shape of the lens by the eye muscles," says Dr. Rapp. "These muscles become tired as the day wears on, especially if they are used by a person who reads all day or does close work."

The strain of reading will be lessened if your posture is correct. The distance between the book and your eyes should be the same as that between your elbow and first knuckles, according to Stuart Clark, O.D., of Reading, Pennsylvania. And reading material should be held or propped at a 20-degree angle from the desk, or if you are standing, at a 10-degree angle.

"Nutrition is also important to your eyes' health," says Dr. Rapp. "You have to keep your whole body healthy to keep your eyes healthy. Eat well, exercise, keep fit and you won't develop eyestrain so readily."

In addition to keeping your eyes healthy, you should give them a rest once in a while. Here are some relaxation techniques.

- Close your eyes for 5 minutes every few hours.
- Look out the window or down the hall about 30 feet. Relax and try to look as broadly as you can, taking in everything, for 30 seconds.
- Hold a pencil at arm's length and pull it slowly toward your eyes until you see double. Repeat for 1 minute a day. This will build your eyes for long-term relief.
- Squeeze your hands together for a few minutes so that the rushing blood makes them warm. Lean back in your chair and cup your palms over your eyes. The heat will relax them.

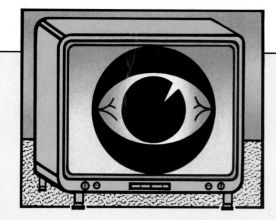

TV without Tired Eyes

Long evenings in front of the television leave many people with tired, red eyes. Stuart Clark, O.D., offers these tips to keep TV-induced eyestrain at a minimum.
- Don't put a lamp on top of your TV. It will cause glare and reduce contrast.
- Sit at least 7 feet away from the set, so that your eyes are level with, or slightly higher than, the set. Never sit so you have to look up at the screen.
- All lighting should come from behind as you watch the set.
- The larger the screen, the better, as long as the picture isn't distorted.

This works even better when performed outside, with the sun's warmth to aid you.

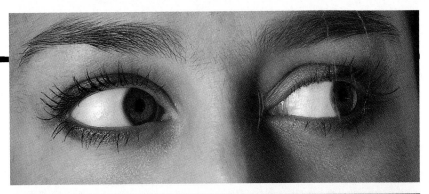

SHEDDING LIGHT ON EYE PROBLEMS

Not all eye muscle fatigue is so simple, however. Your problems can be greatly increased when you spend a lot of time in a place that has improper lighting. One of Dr. Rapp's associates, Alan Lewis, O.D., Ph.D., associate professor of physiological optics, cites three kinds of glare from inadequate lighting that can cause eye fatigue: discomfort glare, disability glare and reflective glare. Discomfort glare is not always immediately apparent, but may cause great fatigue after a while—fluorescent lighting, for example, is often comfortable at first, but not so soothing after a few hours. To test for discomfort glare, enter the room and shield your eyes with a visor or your hand. If the room immediately seems a little more comfortable, discomfort glare is contributing to your eyestrain. To correct the problem, make sure you're sitting so that the light source is to one side, not directly overhead.

Disability glare involves problems with contrast—the difference between light and dark objects, or the letters on a page and the page itself, is muddled. This type of glare is more prevalent among older people, "who need 2 to 2½ times as much contrast as younger people," says Dr. Lewis. So you should increase the quantity of light on the page without increasing the glare. The best way to do this is to rearrange your desk or reading chair so the overhead light falls on your work but doesn't cause shadows.

Reflective glare occurs when glossy paper or a video display unit (VDU) actually reflects a light source into your eyes. The simple solution for this is to put a mirror on your desk where your work usually rests (or set it upright where your VDU is displayed) and move your desk lamp until there is no reflection in the mirror; if the mirror won't

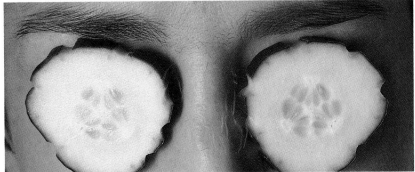

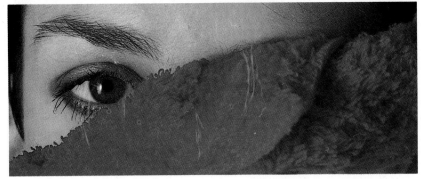

reflect the light source, neither will your paper or screen.

TEARDROP THERAPY

Sometimes eyestrain is caused by a physical problem that has nothing to do with lighting, such as dry eyes. "This is especially a problem for older people," says Joseph Ortiz, M.D., a suburban Philadelphia ophthalmologist. He recommends using "artificial tears," eye drops that can be found in most drugstores, to alleviate the dryness.

Finally, many eyestrain problems are caused by poor vision or diseased eyes. So if the preceding hints don't help relieve your eyestrain, says Dr. Lewis, "get your vision checked thoroughly by a professional. This might be cheaper than running out and ordering new fixtures or having your ceiling torn apart."

For a fast eye refresher: Glance sharply to the left or right corner of your eyes, hold for 30 seconds, then close your eyes and relax for 10 seconds. Repeat, glancing in the other direction. Some other fatigue relievers, which you can place over your eyes, are slices of raw potato or cucumber, cold, moistened tea bags or a cool, damp washcloth.

5

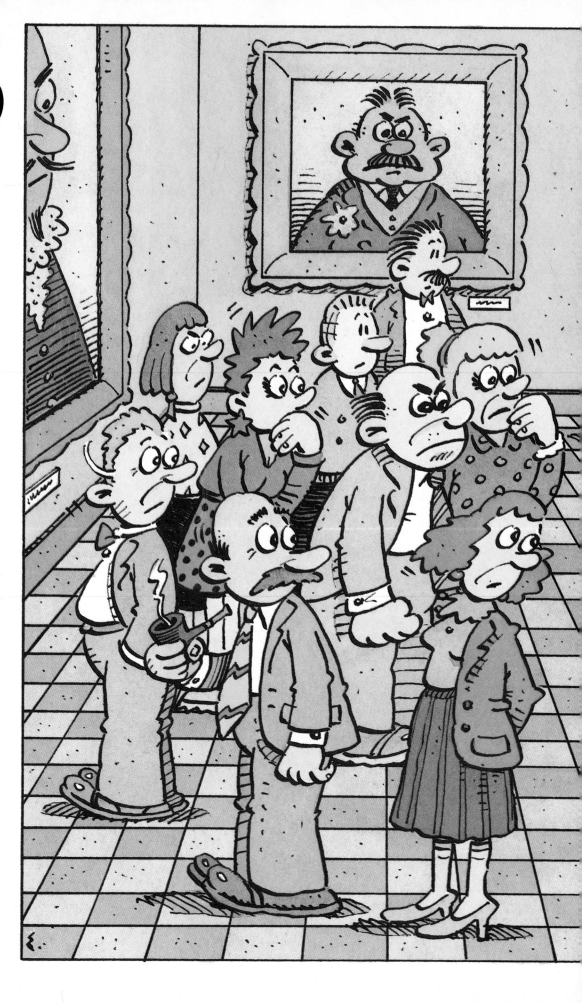

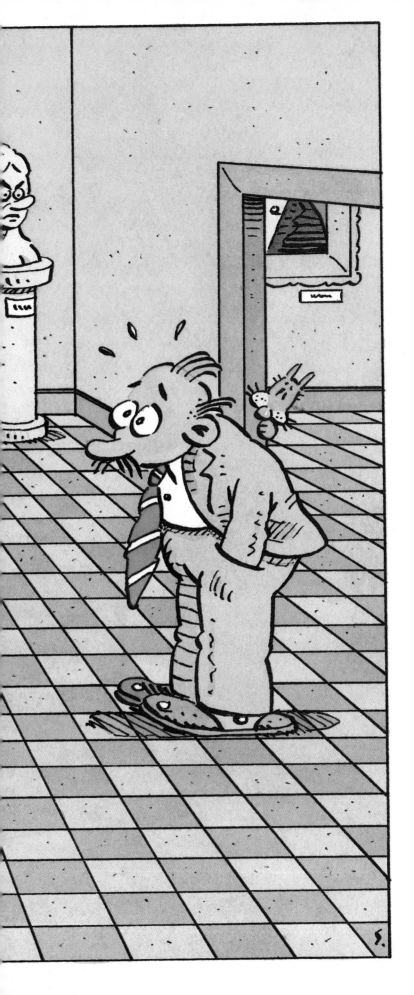

Avoiding Embarrass- ments

You can control the all-too-human sounds, smells and blemishes that make life difficult.

It's happened to all of us. Just when we're closing in on that big contract—or when that special someone looks at us oh-so-lovingly— our body pulls a fast one, emitting offensive sounds or odors.

Being aware of our body means knowing what foods or habits produce these sometimes humiliating reactions, and changing them. If your stomach launches chemical warfare after you eat beans or drink milk, reduce your intake. If your joints crackle like the soundtrack to an old movie when you bend, you're not stretching enough.

But the source of our embarrassment could require more persistent sleuthing. A skin ailment like acne or dandruff could be the result of poor diet, or of a unique pattern of stress and hormones that is curable with vitamins. The agony of hemorrhoids could simply be the result of insufficient fiber in your diet.

Yet no matter how severe or shameful the ailment, it's important to remember that there usually is a physical reason for it, and it can be corrected.

It's rarely necessary to turn to a battery of specialists for even the most mortifying problems like persistent bedwetting. Natural, drug-free treatments that supplement our body's healing powers are within reach for all of us.

When a problem becomes more than a pain in the neck and actually begins to damage your health, like the wearing down of molars by teeth grinding, or insomnia due to snoring so bad it wakes you up, it's best to consult a specialist. But for most of the noisy, smelly or visually unappealing disorders we're all afflicted with, living sensibly is the best solution.

Do you have a problem? Congratulations, you're human.

Snores, Hiccups and Other Body Noises

Our body produces a veritable symphony of sounds, from snaps, crackles and pops to growls, gurgles and roars. Often these noises act as private signals of our body's needs or of some limit to its capacity. But occasionally these announcements go public, greeted perhaps with mirth or disgust. When they do, they become an embarrassment—or even a public nuisance.

Take snoring, for example. Wild West gunfighter John Wesley Hardin was reportedly so upset about a man's snoring that he silenced him with his six-gun. Teddy Roosevelt's nocturnal roars were so loud while he was convalescing in a hospital that his fellow patients nearly instigated a revolt.

What's behind all the ruckus? More men than women snore— the ratio is about five to one—and the evidence seems pretty strong that snoring is related to male hormones, especially testosterone. Snoring is actually caused by obstructions to the free flow of air through the passage at the back of the upper mouth and throat. When this channel is constricted, breathing produces a vibrating noise the same way wind rushing through the reed of a saxophone does—but with considerably less musical effect.

Food allergies, sickness, or structural problems of your nose, mouth or throat can cause snoring. All of these problems are almost invariably correctable. The most common cause is simply poor muscle tone in the throat; 75 percent of snorers are overweight, and the muscles and tissues of their throat are too soft. That's why following a sensible eating and exercise plan should solve most snoring problems. Drinking heavily and taking too many drugs can also over-relax the palate and uvula, so try to avoid them, especially 2 hours before bedtime. Allergies, colds, asthma, deviated septa or respiratory difficulties can also make you snore by obstructing the passage of air through the nose or throat. Try using a humidifier in your bedroom to keep the passages clear, or prop up the head of your bed with two bricks under the front legs to let body fluids drain from your sinuses. If you smoke, quit.

There are more than 300 antisnoring devices on the market today. Be wary about which one you

How Loud Is a Snore?

How would you like to sleep with a yammering jackhammer? Or a ringing alarm clock? If your spouse is in a class with the world's loudest snorers—creating a nightly rumbling of about 80 decibels—you're doing what amounts to the same thing.

In fact, any snorer who exceeds a 75-decibel average during an 8-hour night is overstepping the U.S. Environmental Protection Agency standards for noise pollution, and could seriously impair your hearing.

So if your Prince Charming by day turns into a diesel bus by night, it could be grounds for separation—of your sleeping quarters. You could save your hearing and your marriage.

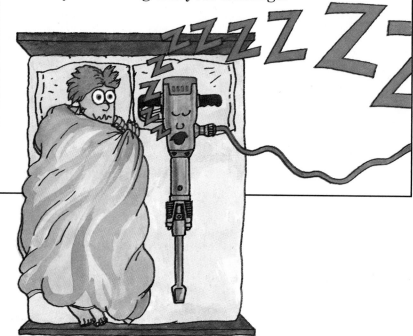

purchase. They range from the harmlessly wacky to the simply sadistic, like the elaborate device that stings you with an electric shock if you snore too loudly. Most snoring starts when a snorer is flat on his back, so a "snore ball"—any rounded object, like a marble or half of a rubber ball— taped or sewed to the loud one's pajamas will stop the snoring, though it might interfere with his sleep.

CRACKING JOINTS

If your back or knees crackle like small-arms fire, don't worry. Cracking relieves excess pressure on the joint. When the muscles surrounding a joint get too tense, they put unequal pressure on it. Cracking just makes the joint looser.

Bones in your knee are actually moving against each other when your knees pop, but most other joints contain a lubricant called synovial fluid. Synovial fluid contains liquid nitrogen, which turns to gas when you crack your joint, the way gas bubbles up in champagne when you pull the cork. Your body is saluting you! It's quite okay to pop your joints when they feel too stiff, but do so in moderation. Otherwise your joints will get too loose.

AIRED GRIEVANCES

If you've ever walked away from a bar with more than just a few joints loose, you know the almost cosmic serenity of letting out a few *basso profundo* belches. They're caused by eating or drinking too fast, and swallowing too much air. The air is then forced upward from the stomach through the throat; world-class burpers produce their sublime sonatas by swallowing air, then expelling it forcibly, using the diaphragm. And if you're ever in that delicate situation where it becomes a dire question of whether to belch or not to belch, go ahead—discreetly, if

possible. Air lodged too long in the stomach can produce a large bubble and aggravate indigestion.

STOMACH GROWLS

A stomach that gurgles like Jacques Cousteau's submarine comes from another intestinal force, fluid or gas under pressure. Our intestines are always busy, moving along air, fluid and solids from the stomach, and when you're too full or too empty, they make that gurgling sound. It's exactly the same principle as an organ pipe, but so far no one's written an aria for stomachs. Your inner stomach contracts when you're hungry and expands when you're full, forcing the contents through at high pressure. Keeping some (healthy) munchies around should solve the contraction problem; leaving the table before you're full should solve the expansion problem.

CURING THE HICCUPS

Another type of bodily faux pas may aggravate you but provide endless mirth for those around you: hiccups. Hiccups are just a muscular response of the diaphragm reacting to off-kilter nerve impulses triggered by eating or drinking too much or too fast. Nobody knows exactly why the nervous system goes on strike like this, but we do know a sure-fire cure, shown in the photo on this page.

If you're in company that would regard the knife-in-the-water trick as some kind of pagan ritual, soak a lemon wedge in angostura bitters and chew it up, rind and all. If the thought of trying *that* makes your taste buds wither, gently rub a cotton swab on the roof of your mouth where the soft palate begins and the hard palate ends, on a point just about in the center of the palate. The light pressure should still your runaway reflexes.

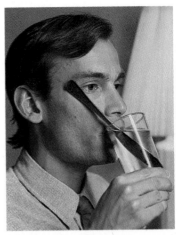

Here's an odd but proven remedy for those uncontrollable hic—the hic—hic— hic—er, singultus, as the medical community calls them. Fill a glass with water and put a metal fork, knife or spoon in it. Then sip the water slowly, holding the upper part of the handle of the utensil against your temple.

Bad Breath, Body Odor and Gas

Bad breath, body odor and strong winds from down under fuel some of the oldest and funniest jokes in the world—until they affect us, that is. Although each of us possesses a unique scent signature, it's important to distinguish normal, minor odors from real social or health problems.

THE GAS CRISIS

Joseph Pujol, a Frenchman known as *le Pétomane* (the Farter), turned his flatulence into very profitable art at the turn of the century, shattering the air of the bawdy Moulin Rouge with his amazing wind instrument.

Le Pétomane was oddly gifted: His music had no odor. For the rest of us who can't rake in 20,000 francs a night after eating beans, flatulence can pose a real problem, medically termed "meteorism."

Though beans have acquired a nasty reputation, it's not the beans themselves that cause flatulence, but the inability of the digestive tract to digest them properly. Gas is produced when the bacteria in the lower bowel begin fermenting foods that have been incompletely absorbed— the way fermenting grapes make champagne. Beans contain complex sugars that our bodies can't break down into smaller sugars that could be absorbed. The result is a spectacular tenfold increase in gas production. There is a way to have your beans and eat them, too. Soak them in water for at least 3 hours, change the water, then boil for at least 30 minutes. There are other dietary culprits besides beans to watch out for; see Hint #12 on page 114 for a list of them.

Stress may cause meteorism, too, because the food moves much faster through your system when you're tense, causing it to be only partially digested and providing the bacteria in your colon with raw material. Try not to eat when you're upset; or if you must, eat slowly or very little until you feel better.

An aerobic activity like jogging will speed up digestion and help eliminate gas but might make things unpleasant for those bringing up the rear. Activated charcoal tablets help, too, acting like a magnet in your system, adsorbing many chemicals, like gas.

A dozen passages of gas a day is normal; anything over that becomes air pollution. If, despite your best efforts, meteorism persists, see a doctor. You could have a pancreatic or gastric disorder. In the meantime, try behavior modification: Avoid crowded elevators during your baked-bean hootenany, or just glare indignantly at the next guy.

NO SWEAT

Stress, heat and exercise all make us sweat, but it isn't the sweat that can knock out a rhinoceros at 50 yards, it's the bacteria that grow in it. There are two kinds of sweat glands designed to keep the body cool: eccrine and apocrine. Eccrine sweat glands are all over the body; apocrine sweat glands are found only in the armpit and genital areas and begin to function during adolescence. There's some truth in the cliché "sweet as a baby"—sexually developed adults perspire more than babies and older people.

Diet can be a factor, too. Garlic, onions and other members of that family can cause objectionable odor when absorbed through the bloodstream and sweated out, but the reeking villain could also be choline-rich foods like eggs, fish, liver and legumes.

Staying clean is the best way to keep friends. Wash with soap frequently, especially around your crotch and armpits. Baking soda, vinegar or talcum powder sprinkled under the arms absorb moisture, while antiperspirant sprays actually stop perspiration (see "Extra-Dry— Or All Wet?").Wearing loose clothing made of natural fibers like cotton allows ventilation and can greatly reduce the amount of perspiration that clings to your body and breeds bacteria. Another trick: Change whatever you use to sweeten your scent every few days. Your body can develop an immunity to one product.

FRESHER BREATH

Almost anything you eat—or smoke or drink—can produce foul odors. Tobacco and coffee are especially notorious halitosis agents.

Mouth odor often starts with a coated tongue, mouldering bits of matter caught between teeth, abscessed teeth, unclean dentures or infections anywhere throughout the respiratory system, from the tonsils to the lungs.

Most cases of killer breath can be cured by a program of good dental hygiene. Brushing after every meal and flossing once a day can only do your breath good: A Kentucky dentist, Michael Lerner, D.M.D., estimates that 95 percent of Americans have soft, inflamed gums that make their breath smell bad.

Joseph Tonzetich, Ph.D., a Canadian dentistry professor, conducted a study in Vancouver to determine the best method of combating the foul breath we wake up to in the morning, and he found brushing the tongue reduced bad breath by 75 percent. Brushing the teeth reduced it by only 25 percent—but the two methods combined reduced it by 85 percent.

Mouthwash, however, is just a cosmetic solution, and a poor one at that. Most mouthwashes contain sugar and alcohol (some are 140 proof!), both of which can cause bad breath. You're entering a vicious circle with mouthwash: The more you use, the more you need. Certain herbs and spices can freshen your breath naturally. Try parsley or cloves, or fennel or anise seeds.

Sweeter Feet

We all know that garlic, onions and peppers cause bad breath, but did you know that these same offenders can also lead to *foot* odors? Although no mouthwash for feet has yet been developed, there are many other precautions that you can take to make sure your feet stay odor free.

Wear shoes that allow your feet to breathe; sandals or shoes made of porous leather or canvas, especially those with open toes, are all good bets. Rubber and plastic shoes trap the ½ pint of moisture that the 250,000 sweat glands in your feet leave in your shoes every day.

You can also wear deodorizing insoles such as Odor Eaters, which contain antibacterial ingredients and activated charcoal to destroy odor and absorb perspiration.

Give yourself a daily foot bath. Use an antibacterial soap to wash between your toes, and when you are done, dry your feet thoroughly. Or soak your feet in a mixture of ½ cup white vinegar to 2 quarts water. This not only kills foot odor, it refreshes your feet as well.

Wear socks made of natural fibers—cotton or cotton blends in the summertime, wool blends during winter. They allow air to reach your feet.

Air out your shoes for at least 24 hours between wearings, giving the moisture in your shoes a chance to evaporate.

Don't use antiperspirants on your feet. The aluminum in such products can cause allergic reactions.

Finally, get enough rest. Tired feet perspire excessively and encourage odor-causing bacterial growth.

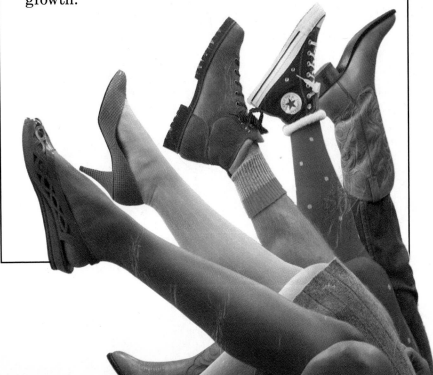

Acne, Dandruff and Liver Spots

If you believe the skin care ads, skin problems fizzle your love life—in fact, the opposite sex won't even enter the same time zone. But when hindrances to our beauty pop up, strict attention to cleanliness, eating and general health habits can conquer most skin problems.

The great exception is acne. *Acne vulgaris*, as common acne is called, is the result of a complex and poorly understood interplay of stress, heredity, diet and hormones.

A hormone called androgen prompts the sebaceous (oil-producing) glands to manufacture sebum, the skin's natural oil, in all of us. Normally, the sebum passes peaceably through the sebaceous ducts and hair follicles to the skin's surface, where it acts as a lubricant for smooth skin. But in acne sufferers, the excess sebum never reaches the surface of the skin; instead, it mixes with bacteria and cells nestled at the base of tiny hair follicles on the face, neck, chest and back, creating a plug that blocks the pore. A closed blemish is called a whitehead, or closed comedone. Although blackheads, or open comedones, may seem more resistant to cleansing, they aren't inflamed, as whiteheads are, and heal more easily.

Although dermatologists have historically pointed an accusing finger at greasy food and germy hands as the cause of acne, the roles of diet and hygiene are now viewed as minimal. Chocolate, for instance, has been completely exonerated. Iodine and animal fats such as milk products have yet to be cleared; their relatively high incidence in the American diet may account for the persistent travelers' reports of more acne in America than in other industrialized nations. People have an enormous range of sensitivity to foods, and if you strongly believe that a particular food causes flare-ups, by all means avoid it.

There are, however, some foods—and individual nutrients—that may be able to help *stop* flareups. Vitamins A and E and zinc, for example, may help clear up *acne vulgaris*. And there's evidence that polyunsaturated oils in the diet can prevent acne explosions. Fish, peanut and vegetable oils may help the sebum flow more easily and prevent clogging.

Unplug Your Pores with Steam

Many salon beauticians give facial steambaths as part of their treatment of acne blemishes. Steam melts the sebum, or oil, that plugs pores, making blackheads easier to extract.

To give yourself a facial steambath, remove any traces of makeup and cleanse your face gently but thoroughly. Then bring a large pot of water to a boil. (If you like, you can add 2 or 3 bags of camomile tea or other aromatic herbs such as peppermint, lavender or rosemary to the water. That makes the steambath doubly pleasant and invigorating.) When the water reaches the boiling point, remove the pot from the heat.

Drape a large, fluffy towel over your head and steam your face for 5 to 10 minutes, leaning no closer than 10 to 12 inches from the water, so you don't scald your skin.

To avoid scarring and infection, be sure that your hands are scrupulously clean and use cotton balls to gently squeeze any blackheads.

Swedish researchers have found that oral zinc supplements of 135 milligrams are as effective as commonly prescribed antibiotics like tetracycline, without the side effects. (This dosage level should be taken only under a doctor's supervision.)

Vitamin A, used successfully in ointment form by dermatologists to normalize skin conditions, has now been modified and used in a very potent oral medication that can cure acne. Accutane, as it is called, is only for the most severe cases; users have reported side effects like dryness of the eyes, chapped lips and even birth defects.

THE DANDRUFF DILEMMA

"Dandruff" is a term applied rather loosely to all flaking scalp conditions, none of which is contagious. Microorganisms on our skin combine with the body's normal secretions of sweat and oil to form a layer that protects the scalp from drying out. Stress, hormonal disturbances and dietary imbalances can kick off a chemical change that alters the scalp's protective layer, lowering its resistance. The normal shedding of skin on the scalp is speeded up, and a substance is secreted that causes the flakes of skin and oil to cling to each other and to the scalp. These oily flakes clog the hair follicles and keep the natural oils from being distributed along the hair shaft.

Hormones and, according to a few physicians, diets high in animal fats, salt and sugar are the leading villains. Stress, allergies to hair products and food allergies may also set off dandruff. Using a mild shampoo daily will help prevent hair follicle clogs. (Zinc pyrithione or selenium sulfide shampoos are the most effective.) A diet rich in fruits, vegetables and grains can also improve the scalp's condition. Fifteen to 20 milligrams of zinc taken daily may be effective, say doctors, because zinc boosts the body's immune system.

Mouthwash—A Dandruff Solution

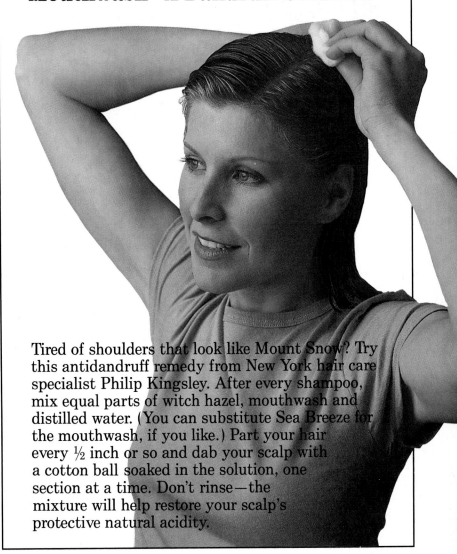

Tired of shoulders that look like Mount Snow? Try this antidandruff remedy from New York hair care specialist Philip Kingsley. After every shampoo, mix equal parts of witch hazel, mouthwash and distilled water. (You can substitute Sea Breeze for the mouthwash, if you like.) Part your hair every ½ inch or so and dab your scalp with a cotton ball soaked in the solution, one section at a time. Don't rinse—the mixture will help restore your scalp's protective natural acidity.

The sun's ultraviolet rays can sometimes reduce dandruff problems. They act as an antiseptic, killing off germs. But too much sun can also aggravate dandruff, causing the tender skin of your scalp to peel. Wearing a lightweight, light-colored hat or scarf will protect your scalp.

SEEING SPOTS

Liver spots, sometimes dubbed age spots or sun spots, have nothing to do with age or stress (or your liver), but are caused by the sun.

The best way to banish blotches is to simply stay out of the sun; if you can't do that, use a broad-spectrum sunscreen or an opaque sunscreen like zinc oxide. Cover your uneven skin tone with makeup designed for the job.

Varicose Veins and Hemorrhoids

Hemorrhoids and varicose veins are part of the high price we pay for civilization, it seems: People in nonindustrial societies rarely have them. Although many people consider them a humiliating, disfiguring nuisance, neither is merely a cosmetic headache. Left untreated, both can become crippling, but both are preventable with one of the most potent "medications" you can buy without a prescription: fiber.

Varicose veins are so common among women over 50 that you're in the minority if you don't suffer from them. The British medical journal *Lancet* reports that varicose veins are "a normal feature of the European body, considerably more common than is red hair or left-handedness."

Despite that sweeping statement, varicose veins are *not* a normal bodily malfunction, and they *are* preventable, although if someone in your family is afflicted, you are likely to get them, too.

What are varicose veins? Simply, veins that have lost their elasticity. The veins in your legs are forced to pump blood 4 or 5 feet up to the heart, fighting gravity all the way. To help make man's evolutionary switch from his four-footed ancestry to walking upright, nature designed ingenious, one-way valves to prevent a backflow of stale, oxygen-depleted blood. Varicose veins occur when these valves break down and the veins lose their elasticity.

The theories on why the veins break down vary considerably. Some researchers blame the strain of sitting or standing too much; others blame constipation and straining to eliminate hard stools, which puts enormous pressure on leg veins. Taking birth control pills may aggravate varicose veins, because these drugs can promote blood clotting. All these explanations point to a defect in circulation, which the dynamic duo of fiber and exercise can help.

Varicose veins are a recurrent problem. Once you've got them, you'll have to keep them under control; switching to a high-fiber diet of whole grains, bran, wheat germ, fresh vegetables and fruit and adhering to a regimen of regular exercise can keep the symptoms at bay. Avoid tight clothing that constricts blood flow, like high boots, too-snug pantyhose, girdles and corsets.

Tight support stockings can help keep the swelling under control, but they're addictive. They will squeeze your legs so tightly that the veins are compressed and blood won't pool. Removing them makes the veins sag again; you can take them off only to sleep.

Your other options are sclerotherapy or surgery. Sclerotherapy can be performed in the doctor's office; he drains the offending vein of blood, then injects it with a hardening agent that forms an artificial blood clot and effectively kills the vein. The failure rate is

Getting the Jump on Varicose Veins

The best way to shake varicose veins is to *move*! Doctors from the Mayo Clinic in Rochester, Minnesota, say walking lowers the pressure in your veins to a *third* of what it is when you are standing.

Avoid long periods of sitting and standing. If you must be inactive, flex your leg muscles, wiggle your toes and slowly raise and lower yourself on the balls of your feet. Don't cross your legs; that cuts off the circulation. On long plane, bus or train rides, pace up and down the aisle at least once an hour. If you sit all day at work, elevate your feet 12 to 24 inches above the level of your heart whenever you can; that reduces pressure in the veins to almost zero.

Walking, jogging, cycling and swimming improve your circulation and the muscle tone in your legs. Take brisk 15-minute walks 4 times a day if you can. Going barefoot around the house helps exercise foot muscles and improves venous blood flow, too.

high, and the procedure injures the vein valves. Surgery is much simpler: The veins are simply stripped away. But if you desire surgery just to make your legs more alluring, you could be in for a disappointment: If the skin has become discolored, surgery won't help.

THE ONE-INCH ITCH

Hemorrhoids affect at least 50 percent of adults of both sexes over the age of 50 and get more common as people age. One researcher goes so far as to say that there's not a woman alive who doesn't have them if she's given birth.

Hemorrhoids might never be acceptable cocktail chatter, but they're nothing to be ashamed of. A British researcher describes them as caused simply by a downward displacement of the anal canal lining. There is some 25 feet of digestive tract in the human body, and hemorrhoids affect only the last inch or so. Simply, these unpleasant little visitors are swollen veins inside or outside the rectum.

Hemorrhoids can be brought almost completely under control with one of the cheapest preparations around: fiber. In a Danish study, 84 percent of patients with hemorrhoids who were fed fiber daily showed improvement, and 69 percent said they still had fewer symptoms *three months later.*

Fiber not only can prevent hemorrhoids, but it's likely that it plays an important role in relieving them. Among its other jobs, fiber helps push waste out of the bowel before it forms the hard stools that irritate hemorrhoidal tissue; a diet high in refined foods may cause the hard stools and induce constipation.

It's easier to introduce fiber into your life than you might think; it's found in most fruits and vegetables, grains and cereals. Try to eat a variety of these foods, and drink plenty of water to keep the stools soft. Avoid excessive coffee,

Three Ways to Avoid Hemorrhoid Surgery

Doctors consider hemorrhoidectomies—the surgical removal of hemorrhoids—to be very effective. But the immense pain, 3- to 5-day hospital stay and weeks of bedrest that follow keep it from being the treatment of choice for many hemorrhoid sufferers. Fortunately, doctors have developed new procedures that cut down the pain and inconvenience.

In *rubber band ligation,* a rubber band is shot around a swollen vein with a specially constructed gun. The band strangles the vein, killing it. This virtually painless procedure can be performed in the doctor's office and doesn't require anesthesia.

Cryodestruction uses a nitrous oxide probe to isolate and destroy hemorrhoids by freezing them. The treatment is uncomfortable but not painful enough to require sedation.

Dilatation, or stretching of the anal canal, was pioneered by doctors who believe that swollen veins are caused by straining against a too-tightly contracted anal muscle band. Patients undergoing dilatation are anesthetized for a short time, during which the anal canal is widely dilated. Patients follow up by using a special dilator at home.

tea, cola or alcohol; they irritate the bowel.

Toilet habits can aggravate hemorrhoids by increasing the pressure on your legs and backside. Try resting your heels on a small bench when enthroned; that's closer to the natural squatting position.

Like their cousins varicose veins, hemorrhoids are chronic. Fortunately, hemorrhoids need not mean constant pain, and there are a number of measures you can take to control any discomfort. To avoid further irritation, wipe with a wet cloth instead of toilet paper; better yet, rinse gently with warm water. To soothe the maddening itch, dab gently with witch hazel wipes, available in any drugstore. Alternating hot-water baths with ice packs will relieve the pain. Over-the-counter preparations offer temporary relief of symptoms that could subside naturally within 48 hours.

Never assume bleeding from the colon is just a hemorrhoid: It could be something as serious as colon cancer.

Bedwetting, Sleepwalking and Nighttime Tooth Grinding

Night is when all our darkest, most primeval fears assault us, when we lapse into the deepest, most hidden recesses of our mind during sleep. Perhaps that's why we feel so mystified by such nighttime phenomena as bedwetting, sleepwalking and tooth grinding (or bruxism, as doctors call it). But there's no reason to stay in the dark. Current research has shed new light on these problems.

Take bruxism, for example. Once explained by Freudians as a nocturnal release of bottled-up aggression, it is now viewed as the product of stress, poor nutrition, allergies, or simply physical problems of the lower jaw. We'll look at jaw problems first.

Dentists and researchers have lumped all lower jaw problems into the tongue-twisting category of Temporomandibular Joint Disorder (TMJ).

The lower jaw differs from most other paired parts of the human body. Your left foot can move while the right one stays still; but if the muscles, joints, bones and tendons on both sides of your jaw fail to mesh perfectly, a host of health problems can set in, with bruxism among them.

To correct this jaw problem, some dentists file down the teeth or use muscle relaxant drugs. But many are leaning toward prescribing a clear plastic mouth guard like the ones used by football players. Fortunately, your "game time" is only at night. One dentist claims this device works for 80 percent of his bruxing patients, who usually have to wear it for three to six months.

More children brux than adults; as many as 20 percent of all children grind their teeth at night. That may be due to the perpetual emotional and physical changes they go through as they grow, but there are other reasons as well. If your child is allergic to something, there is a 60 percent chance he bruxes, according to one Miami researcher.

If allergies cause you or your child to brux at night, try to relieve the allergic symptoms. Or add calcium to the diet. A study in which bruxing patients increased their calcium intake showed a dramatic decline in nighttime grinding. Calcium, found in milk products and fish, helps build healthy bones and keeps muscles and nerves—all of which are involved in making the lower jaw work—in top condition.

WETNESS WOES

Consistently wet sheets have probably prompted even more quack cures than baldness. But today's verdict is unanimous: Childhood bedwetting is almost certainly caused by an immature nervous system. Bedwetting happens to every one of us when we are babies; the nervous system hasn't gotten around to controlling the bladder yet. Fifteen percent of all five-year-olds wet their beds, according to one estimate. The problem is probably inherited; if you wet your bed when you were a child, chances are 77 percent that your child will, too. Some of us mature more slowly than others; the almost unimaginably complex structure called the nervous system must mature, too. Time, patience and an understanding attitude are the best solutions.

Yet allergies might be at fault here as well. A study conducted between 1956 and 1979, involving 600 children who wet their beds, found 60 percent did so because they were allergic to cow's milk. (Other likely foods were eggs, chocolate, grains and citrus fruits.) Just as sinus passages can become swollen by allergies, so can the passages running to and from the bladder, resulting in a loss of that distinctive pinching sensation that signals your bladder is full. The child doesn't feel that the bladder is full at night, and voids without waking.

Sometimes the problem has a mechanical basis, such as an obstruction of the urethra. Your doctor may wait until the child is approaching adolescence before proceeding with costly tests.

Quick cures range from high-tech—an alarm that goes off when the child voids or stimulants to keep him awake—to homey. One ex-bedwetter recalled that his British nanny came up with an impeccably efficient solution: She gave him a large glass of water just before bedtime, then woke him up an hour after he fell asleep to go to the bathroom.

MOONLIGHT STROLLS

Contrary to popular belief, sleepwalking is not a way to act out dreams—it occurs in the nondream stage of sleep. And in children, at least, it has nothing to do with subconscious struggles.

Sleepwalking develops in 10 to 15 percent of all children, and like bedwetting, is probably the result of an immature nervous system. In fact, sleepwalkers wet their beds more frequently than other children, and the two seem to be connected. Here, too, the cure is a capsule of time.

Although children who sleepwalk should *never* be treated as if they have emotional problems, adult sleepwalking is a different story. In adults this problem is clearly stress related and may be a symptom of a deeper disorder. If the sleepwalker and his family aren't disturbed by a few incidents, it's best to leave the sleepwalker alone. But if the sleepwalker starts to wander ever farther afield, some form of psychotherapy should be considered.

A new theory says sleepwalking stems from a lack of serotonin in the bloodstream. (Serotonin is one of the brain's chemical messengers.) A study at Rutgers University Medical School showed that 30 percent of a group of 60 children with migraine headaches sleepwalked, about nine times more than children without migraines. The researchers say that

migraines and sleepwalking could be symptoms of the same disorder—serotonin deficiency—and could be eliminated by raising serotonin levels. (Altering serotonin levels is easier than it sounds: An essential amino acid called tryptophan, found in many protein foods like milk, turkey, whole grains and beans, stimulates the brain's production of serotonin.)

Probably the most important part of dealing with sleepwalking is ensuring that the sleepwalker doesn't hurt himself. Remove all objects he could trip over, lock windows and doors and follow him to make sure he doesn't get into trouble. It's not dangerous to awaken a sleepwalker, despite popular belief, but the sleepwalker could be quite shocked to wake up, say, on a diving board, so wake him as gently as you would any sleeper.

Home Remedies for Bedwetting

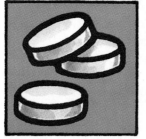

Bedwetting can be one of life's most embarrassing health problems—and one of the most difficult to solve. But some readers of *Prevention* magazine have written the publication to say that certain home reme-dies have worked for members of their families.

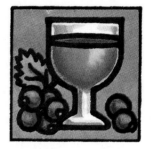

One grandparent swears by calcium: "Our grandson, 5, stopped wetting the bed immediately after we gave him calcium tablets—first 3 a day, now 1 after lunch and 1 before bedtime."

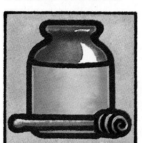

A parent wrote: "Our youngest girl had wet the bed every night of her 9 years. When she developed a problem I took her to a chiropractor, who suggested 4 ounces of cranberry juice a day. That night she slept dry."

And several letters have come in claiming that a spoonful of honey given at bedtime is an answer to bedwetting problems.

6

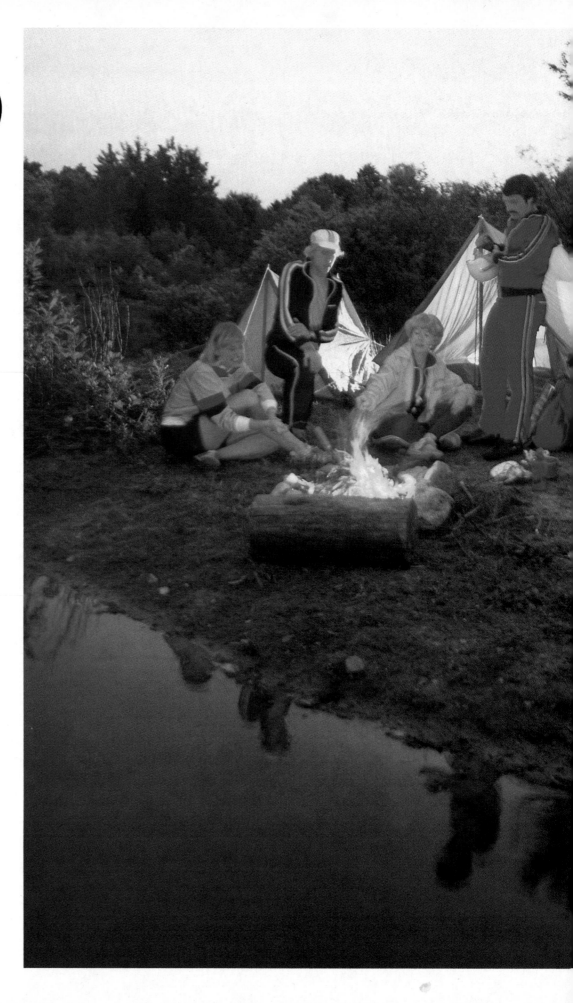

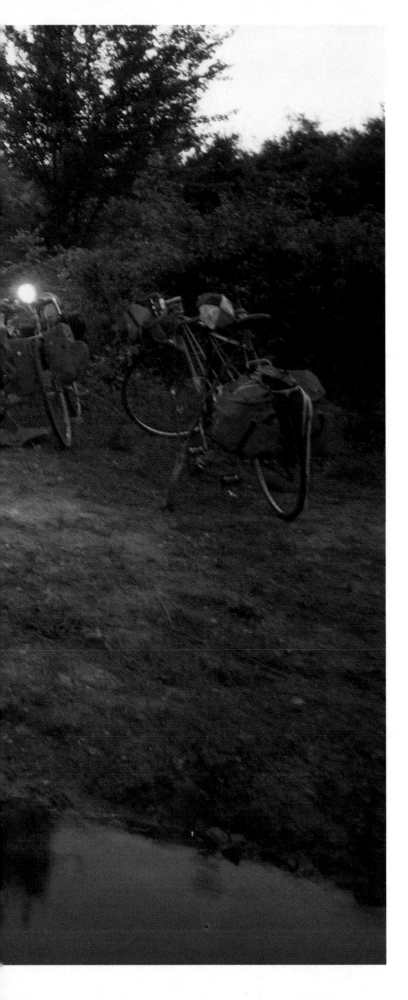

Enjoying Travel and the Outdoors

How to keep your vacations and leisure time healthy, safe and worry free.

From 1979 to 1982, a small party led by Sir Ranulph Twistleton-Wykenham Fiennes and his wife, Lady Virginia, traveled on the first transglobe expedition, which took them from their home in England to Antarctica and then to the North Pole. Traveling by ship, rubber raft, aluminum canoe and snowmobile, they had to cope with lizards and bats, fatigue, intense freezing conditions and a fire that destroyed their supplies. When they reached the South Pole, their halfway point, seven weeks ahead of schedule, they celebrated with a game of cricket.

Few of us will ever have to endure these travelers' travails, yet all of us have something in common with Sir Ranulph and friends every time we travel: a sense of adventure tempered by the desire to minimize the hazards of roughing it.

Now, a transglobe expedition isn't everyone's idea of vacation adventure. Perhaps you'd prefer idling in a French cafe or hopping a flight to Las Vegas. Or maybe your idea of relaxation is to loll on a beach somewhere, camp in some piney mountains, or just putter in your backyard.

No matter what form your idea of leisure pleasure takes, leaving the shelter of home always makes us vulnerable to nature's vagaries. The key to enjoying your time away from home is to feel you still have some control over your health, safety and the basic comforts, despite nature's dice rolls.

Whether your biggest vacation nemesis is poison ivy or motion sickness, frostbite or fear of flying, you'll find practical guidance here. Next time you're feeling at two with nature, turn to these pages.

Motion Sickness and Turista

Jane's friend Chris drove like a New York City cabbie, with sudden, jerky thrusts each time she shifted gears. Jane needed this lift to the bank, but within 5 minutes she felt dizzy, sweaty and nauseated. If only she could get out of the car and breathe fresh air!

Researchers don't fully understand why some people, like Jane, experience motion sickness while others never do. It is known, however, that the illness results when motion causes shifts in the canals of the inner ear. When such shifts occur, our equilibrium can be thrown off. Certain factors aggravate motion sickness—riding in a hot, stuffy car, riding backward or watching the horizon lurch up and down.

Researchers now theorize that the cause of motion sickness can be found in the conflict between motion as sensed by the eye and as perceived by the inner ear's balance receptors, says Mike Samuels, M.D. You can put this principle to work for you quite simply.

Since back-seat riders tend to suffer more than front-seat riders, you should sit in the front seat and aim your eyes above the horizon by about 45 degrees to nullify the effects of a visually bouncing horizon. If your children get carsick, they'll often feel better if you get them to lie down, close their eyes and keep their head still. Or they can sit in the front seat, keeping their eyes focused out the front window in the direction the car is heading (not out the sides or back).

If you get airsick, you can curb queasiness by flying at night, when there is little visual stimulation. It also helps to sit away from the engines or near the plane's center of gravity.

Drugs like Dramamine or Marezine are traditionally prescribed for motion sickness and are effective for 4 to 6 hours. For longer relief, doctors can now prescribe a dime-size patch that you can stick on the skin behind your ear. The patch contains an antinausea drug called scopolamine that trickles through the skin and into the body over a 72-hour period. This drug does have some side effects, however. One pharmacist reported that when she placed the patch behind her left ear, the vision in her left eye became blurred, her pupil enlarged and her mouth became very dry. (See "Ginger Root for the Road" for an effective nondrug preventive.)

TURISTA: TRIP SPOILER

Travelers warned to watch out for bugs would probably think of the large crawly type native to the tropics. But another bug bothers many who journey to faraway places—traveler's diarrhea, or "turista," as it is popularly known. This short-term but troublesome disorder affects an estimated 40 percent of those who travel to developing countries. While it has many causes, it is most often believed to be due to the bacteria *Escherichia coli*, which proliferates in food and water.

Some simple precautions could

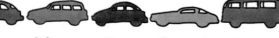

Ginger Root for the Road

Ginger may outperform common drugstore remedies as a cure for motion sickness. In a study of 36 college students prone to motion sickness, psychologists gave dimenhydrinate (Dramamine) to one group, a placebo to a second group and 2 gelatin capsules of powdered ginger root to a third. Each student was then blindfolded and given a 6-minute ride on a revolving chair. Both the dimenhydrinate and the placebo group felt nauseated and had to stop before the time was up. Half of the ginger root group stayed the course the entire 6 minutes without discomfort.

The researchers speculated that Dramamine, an antihistamine, works by making the brain *think* the stomach's not upset, while the powdered ginger root helps your stomach directly by absorbing acids and blocking stomach upset.

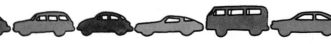

mean the difference between spending your vacation running to the bathroom or to the beach. Start by avoiding the tap water unless you know for sure that it passes through an efficient purification plant. Unfortunately, most short-term travelers have no easy way to determine how pure the water is. Just to be safe, it's best to drink water or other beverages that have been bottled, making sure that they have been well sealed. Don't forget to stick to bottled water for brushing your teeth, as well. If you can't get bottled water, you can sterilize your water supply by boiling it for 10 minutes or by adding special water purification tablets from a drugstore.

Choosing safe foods also requires careful strategy. Eat only well-cooked dishes. Say no to fresh, raw vegetables, food from street vendors and ice in your drinks. Also avoid cold meat, custards, mayonnaise and shellfish in areas where refrigeration could be questionable. When it comes to fruits, eat only those peeled in your presence.

There is a readily available source of information on the safest and most sanitary places to eat and stay—the airlines. Airlines take extra care in choosing lodging for their crews, since a staff epidemic of turista could prove costly and disruptive. Call the airline and inquire where the crew members stay.

If, despite your precautions, turista strikes, you should flush the bacteria with plenty of bottled or boiled water. Liquid clay binders like Kaopectate and prescription drugs like Lomotil can aggravate your condition: By acting as a plug, they keep the bacteria in your system longer. Use them only as an emergency measure until you can see a doctor.

You can also try less costly but equally effective natural remedies. "Activated charcoal is an excellent remedy for traveler's diarrhea," says Marjorie Baldwin, M.D., of the Wildwood Sanitarium and Hospital in Wildwood, Georgia. Follow the dosage instructions on the bottle. The activated charcoal stifles bacteria in the intestines.

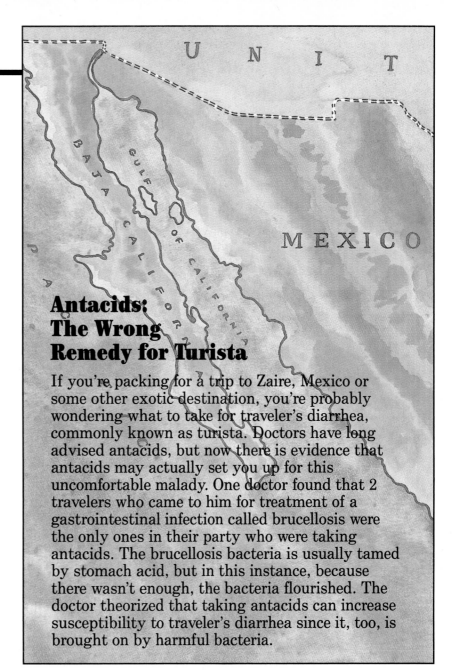

Antacids: The Wrong Remedy for Turista

If you're packing for a trip to Zaire, Mexico or some other exotic destination, you're probably wondering what to take for traveler's diarrhea, commonly known as turista. Doctors have long advised antacids, but now there is evidence that antacids may actually set you up for this uncomfortable malady. One doctor found that 2 travelers who came to him for treatment of a gastrointestinal infection called brucellosis were the only ones in their party who were taking antacids. The brucellosis bacteria is usually tamed by stomach acid, but in this instance, because there wasn't enough, the bacteria flourished. The doctor theorized that taking antacids can increase susceptibility to traveler's diarrhea since it, too, is brought on by harmful bacteria.

Carob flour, often used as a chocolate substitute, can help normalize loose bowels. It's very rich in pectin, which acts as a binding substance. Similarly, bananas, also rich in pectin, have been a traditional fighter against diarrhea. Bananas are rich in potassium, magnesium and other nutrients that diarrhea drains from the body.

Bran can also help fight diarrhea. That's because fiber normalizes the functioning of the intestinal tract. By absorbing water and forming soft bulk, bran will thicken loose, watery stools. Just a few tablespoons followed by a glass of water should help within a couple of days.

Jet Lag and Altitude Sickness

As president, Lyndon Johnson demanded that all his meetings, no matter where in the U.S. they were to be held, be scheduled according to Washington, D.C., time. Johnson wasn't just being stubborn; he simply wanted to be in tip-top mental and physical shape for the demands of the presidency. He couldn't afford to fall prey to "jet lag," the out-of-sync feeling that overcomes you when your plane has landed in San Francisco but your body acts as though it's still in Pittsburgh.

Jet lag happens when your usual schedule of sleep, meals, activity and rest is disrupted. You begin to feel sluggish, drowsy and irritable. Sometimes nervousness, insomnia and indigestion set in.

Few people have LBJ's power to call all the shots, but you can avert jet lag with a few simple strategies.

Harmon Brown, M.D., a member of the U.S. Olympic Committee's Sports Medicine Council, recommends flying to your destination early so you'll have time to adjust. (It usually takes about a day per time zone for your body to readjust.) If you can't leave early, try this the night before you leave: Go to bed about an hour earlier than usual if you're headed east; retire an hour later if you're headed west. Then during the flight, reset your watch to coincide with the time at your destination and readjust your habits accordingly. Once on board the plane, try to stick to the light and darkness cycle of your destination.

A DIET TO BEAT JET LAG

Charles Ehret, Ph.D., senior scientist in the division of biological and

Help for the Fearful Flyer

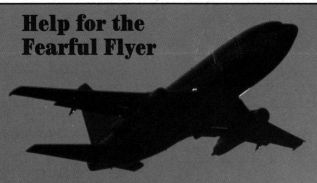

Lisa doesn't like to fly—at least that's what she says. She claims that the hassles of tickets, airport traffic and baggage aren't worth the bother. But Lisa isn't being honest. The truth is that she's *scared* to fly.

Today help is available for Lisa and the 25 million other adults in the U.S. who share her fear. Several programs have been created expressly to teach people how to spread their wings without being afraid to leave the ground. One of the most successful is The Program for the Fearful Flyer, developed by retired Pan American Airways captain T. W. Cummings.

Capt. Cummings travels around the country to run seminars consisting of 4 3-hour meetings, the last held aboard a parked jet. Participants also work with a taped program, which they use to reduce anxiety both before and during a flight.

Participants learn to work through their phobia in 4 steps: mustering the motivation to conquer the fear; understanding the fear; honestly dealing with it; then simulating a flight.

Capt. Cummings also teaches how an airplane works and gives airplane safety statistics (which are a lot more comforting than those for automobiles).

Finally, he accompanies participants on a short graduation flight (not included in the $235 program cost).

Since the program began in 1978, over 3,000 fearful flyers have earned their wings. If you would like to join their ranks, contact the Phobia Society of America, 6110 Executive Boulevard, Rockville, MD 20852 (301-231-9350).

medical research at the U.S. Department of Energy's Argonne National Laboratory, has put together a three-step diet to overcome jet lag that works on a feast/fast cycle. Feasting means eating generous portions, while fasting calls for limiting daily calorie intake to about 700 to 800 calories. The program is based on evidence that the body's inner clocks are regulated by various cycles that are influenced by cues such as darkness and light, the foods you eat and patterns of physical activity. Dr. Ehret says that during the fasting part of the diet the body can be readily reset to a different timetable.

The diet works like this. Set aside one predeparture day for each time zone you'll cross. If you're crossing three zones, for example, begin three days ahead.

The first day is a "feast" day. Stress eggs, cheese, milk or fish for breakfast and lunch to get plenty of protein. Eat lots of complex carbohydrates at supper to help you sleep.

The next day you can still eat protein for breakfast and lunch, but cut the portions in half. Keep carbohydrates and calories to a minimum. Soups and salads are great for these light-meal days. The day of your flight should be a "fast" day.

It's also a good idea to avoid alcohol once you're aboard the plane, since it promotes fatigue and dehydration. Drink lots of liquids, especially juices and water, to replenish the fluids you lose in pressurized plane cabins.

ALTITUDE SICKNESS

In its mild form, altitude sickness means headache or fatigue. In its acute form it can mean nausea, loss of appetite, insomnia, flulike lethargy and breathing difficulties. Problems usually start at 8,000 feet or more above sea level, where the air begins to thin markedly so there is less oxygen. The older you get, the higher your risk of severe symptoms, though people who are moderately active and whose medical problems are well in hand

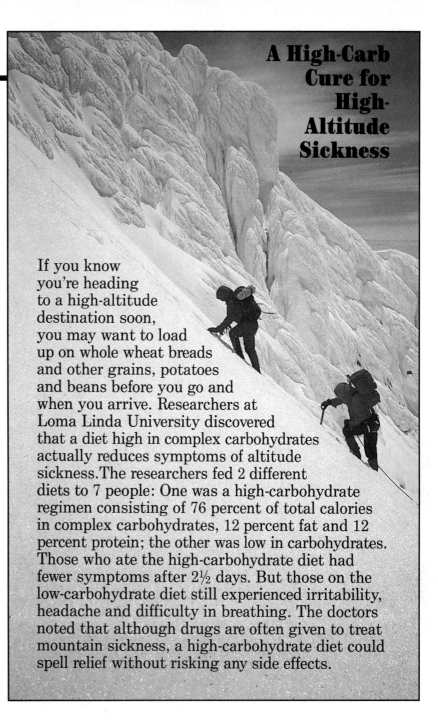

A High-Carb Cure for High-Altitude Sickness

If you know you're heading to a high-altitude destination soon, you may want to load up on whole wheat breads and other grains, potatoes and beans before you go and when you arrive. Researchers at Loma Linda University discovered that a diet high in complex carbohydrates actually reduces symptoms of altitude sickness. The researchers fed 2 different diets to 7 people: One was a high-carbohydrate regimen consisting of 76 percent of total calories in complex carbohydrates, 12 percent fat and 12 percent protein; the other was low in carbohydrates. Those who ate the high-carbohydrate diet had fewer symptoms after 2½ days. But those on the low-carbohydrate diet still experienced irritability, headache and difficulty in breathing. The doctors noted that although drugs are often given to treat mountain sickness, a high-carbohydrate diet could spell relief without risking any side effects.

generally have little to worry about.

Charles Houston, M.D., of the University of Vermont's Program of Environmental Studies, advises even healthy individuals to avoid use of oral contraceptives, sedatives and tranquilizers at high altitudes. Minimize the amount of alcohol, caffeine or other stimulants you drink. To prevent acute mountain sickness, Dr. Houston advises drinking extra fluids and avoiding strenuous activity. If you feel very sick, try complete bed rest for a few days. One sure cure you can always fall back on is to descend a few thousand feet.

Bites, Stings and Rashes

If you've ever been on a camping trip and been assaulted by black flies or watched your legs break out in a mini-mountain range from a brush with poison ivy, you know well the agony of summer's ecstasy: bites, stings and plant allergies.

For many people, insect attacks and poison plants cause only momentary discomfort—a slight prick of pain or an itchy red welt, bothersome today but soon forgotten. If you're allergic to insect venom or to poison plants, however, your reaction can be much more severe, and in rare instances, even life-threatening.

Here's some helpful advice to pack along with your camping gear.

ARMED ATTACKERS

Generally speaking, there are two types of pests that can zap you— stingers and biters. The stingers include hornets, wasps, honeybees and yellow jackets. Biters include

How to Remove a Stinger

Although honeybee stings don't seem to hurt any more than those of yellow jackets, hornets or wasps, they do pose one more problem: They leave the stinger behind. (The weapons of the other pests aren't barbed.)

So what do you do for a honeybee sting? Apply an ice cube to reduce the swelling and numb the pain, then try to flick the stinger out with your fingernail. You might also try to scrape it out with a dull knife. Don't pull at the stinger with tweezers or anything else. You risk squeezing it, which will only force more venom into the wound.

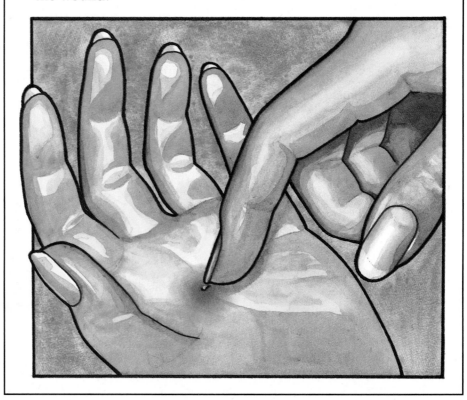

ants, ticks, mosquitoes, spiders and flies. If you've been stung, you should remove the stinger at once (see "How to Remove a Stinger), then thoroughly wash the spot with soap and water. A paste of water and baking soda can reduce itching. Ice can numb pain and itching as well. Two other ingredients right off your kitchen shelf can help, too—fresh lemon or raw onion. To neutralize the toxins of a bee sting, apply a paste of meat tenderizer and water.

Stings on the face, nose, throat or mouth merit medical attention, since swelling in these areas can interfere with breathing or lead to other serious complications.

If you've been bitten, apply an antiseptic to the spot; most bugs that bite have poor reputations for cleanliness.

ALLERGIC REACTIONS

Some people are allergic to insect or spider venom. Their severe reaction, known as anaphylactic shock, can be life-threatening (see "Preparing for Allergic Emergencies"). How can you predict whether you'll be allergic? First, the more venom you get in the sting, the greater the chance of an allergic reaction. Venom levels also vary with the seasons. Honeybees, for instance, carry far less venom in late fall than they do in the peak of summer. In addition, anyone who is allergic to honeybees is likely to be allergic to wasps, yellow jackets, ants and hornets. Also, nearly one-third of people who are allergic to insects are also allergic to drugs, especially those that are injected, like penicillin.

Your body will probably waste little time telling you if it's allergic to bites or stings. Watch for any or all of the following signs of an allergy.

- Severe swelling, not only at the sting area but in other places such as the eyes, lips and tongue
- Dizziness, weakness or collapse
- Widespread itching or hives
- Stomach cramps

Preparing for Allergic Emergencies

Venomous insect stings are the second most common cause of anaphylaxis, a form of shock caused by allergic reactions. If you or a member of your family has ever experienced this life-threatening reaction or has a history of severe allergy symptoms, you should be well pre- pared for a recurrence. The life-savers you'll need are an emergency kit of allergy drugs and an identification bracelet or tag.

The kits are sold at drugstores by prescription. They contain a vial of adrenaline to restore blood pressure and breathing to normal. They also contain antihistamines to shut off the body's release of the substances that trigger the reaction. Many kits also include tourniquets to prevent the spread of venom. Carry one kit in your bag, briefcase or car; leave the other at home.

The I.D. bracelets or tags will save precious time and prevent medical personnel from mistakenly treating you for other causes of collapse. You can order them from Medic Alert Foundation International, P.O. Box 1009, Turlock, CA 95381-1009.

- Nausea or vomiting
- Anxiety
- Bluish skin
- Pain lasting more than 48 hours

If you experience any of these symptoms, seek medical attention immediately. In the meantime, it's important to treat allergic reactions promptly while you're awaiting medical help.

Watch for any signs that the reaction has spread to other parts of your body, especially redness and swelling.

If the bite or sting is on a limb, elevate it to reduce the swelling, and apply ice. Don't apply tourniquets or try to suck venom from the wound.

EENSY WEENSY TROUBLE

Two insect pests are more venomous than all the rest: the black widow and the brown recluse spider. If you

The Four Faces of Poison Ivy

We all learn that poison ivy has 3 shiny leaves on each stem, but there's more to identifying this plant than looking for the telltale threesome. Did you know that poison ivy can grow as a plant, bush or vine? Or that it bears flowers and fruit? Also, poison ivy is toxic all year 'round, even after the leaves have dropped. Below are some season-by-season tips on identifying the plant on sight.

If you're still confused by the visual cues, here's a sure-fire test for poison ivy: Grasp a leaf with a folded piece of paper and crush it with a rock. If the plant in question is poison ivy, the sap released will turn dark brown in 10 minutes and black in a day.

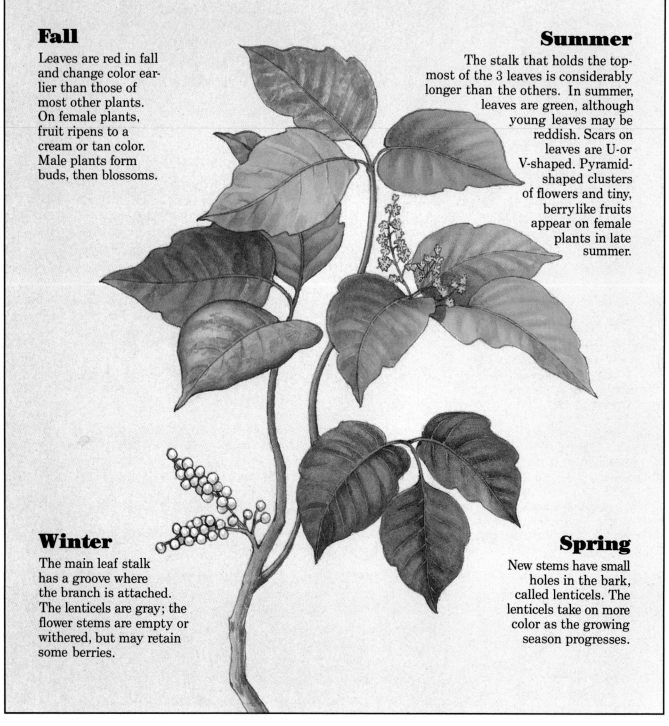

Fall

Leaves are red in fall and change color earlier than those of most other plants. On female plants, fruit ripens to a cream or tan color. Male plants form buds, then blossoms.

Summer

The stalk that holds the topmost of the 3 leaves is considerably longer than the others. In summer, leaves are green, although young leaves may be reddish. Scars on leaves are U-or V-shaped. Pyramid-shaped clusters of flowers and tiny, berrylike fruits appear on female plants in late summer.

Winter

The main leaf stalk has a groove where the branch is attached. The lenticels are gray; the flower stems are empty or withered, but may retain some berries.

Spring

New stems have small holes in the bark, called lenticels. The lenticels take on more color as the growing season progresses.

have been bitten by either of these, don't wait for symptoms to appear. Get to a doctor or hospital emergency room immediately.

The black widow can be identified by the red hourglass-shaped marking on the underside of its shiny black body. A brown recluse spider, also called a fiddler spider, has a distinct, brown, violin-shaped marking on the front portion of its body. Many brown spiders appear similar, so, if possible, kill the critter that bit you and take it to the doctor for identification.

The best way to avoid any kind of spider bite is to wear gloves whenever you have to handle old piles of lumber, rocks or scrap. Destroy spiderwebs with a broom and burn any nests of spider egg sacs that you discover. Stacks of rubbish and dirt are prime hiding places for spiders, so keep them from accumulating in your home, shed, garage or any areas where children play.

FENDING OFF OTHER PESTS

You needn't feel at the mercy of crawling or flying attackers. Commercial insect repellents work fairly well and come in several forms. The main drawback of aerosols is that they are highly flammable and can explode if you leave them too near a campfire, on the sunny dashboard of your car or near another heat source. Nonaerosol versions, such as liquid chemical repellent, are somewhat safer. Some of the formulas smell pretty foul; others have been scented to make them smell more pleasant to humans, but the fragrances can actually attract some insects.

A simpler and less hazardous alternative to chemical repellents is plain citronella oil, derived from a wild grass. Available at pharmacies, citronella oil works just as well as the chemical repellents—and costs far less. You can also buy citronella-scented candles to burn on the patio or at the picnic area.

Another natural repellent is probably sitting on your vitamin shelf: thiamine (vitamin B_1). If you know you'll be in a buggy place, you may want to take a 100-milligram tablet before leaving home. And if you'll be camping, hiking or playing outside for extended periods, consider taking a 100-milligram tablet two to three times a day. When you take such large amounts of thiamine, your body excretes part of the excess through your perspiration. Thiamine's odor may repel insects, but you won't be able to smell a thing. (You should take this level of thiamine for only a few days, and then only with a doctor's okay.)

It also helps to wear light-colored clothing, such as khaki, with long pants and sleeves so that as little skin as possible is exposed. Bright-colored clothing attracts bees, since it looks like flowers. If you can, eliminate damp, marshy or watery areas around your home, which make great breeding grounds for mosquitoes. Be especially careful around garbage cans or rotting fruit under trees. Both are favorite landing strips for honeybees, yellow jackets and wasps. If bees do suddenly buzz around you, don't swat at them or flail your arms. Simply walk away slowly.

Overexposure

Vitamin C and Prickly Heat

Vitamin C may be an effective treatment for prickly heat, the pimply-looking heat rash that itches like crazy. During World War II, Robert L. Stern, M.D., successfully treated American troops suffering from prickly heat in the South Pacific with 300 to 500 milligrams of C a day. Later, British dermatologist T. C. Hindson, M.D., found vitamin C effective for children. In one study, he gave 15 children various dosages of vitamin C, adjusted to each child's weight. The rash improved or disappeared entirely in 14 of them. He believes that vitamin C works by taking over the role of an important enzyme system that keeps our sweat glands from becoming overworked.

J ohn jogged every day with the fanatacism of an evangelical preacher; running was his saving grace. His doctor had warned John, a 49-year-old salesman, that unless he started getting some good, regular exercise, he was a prime candidate for a heart attack. So he jogged daily—6, 7, even 10 miles. And he didn't cut back on his routine despite the searing heat wave that had come over his hometown in Nebraska.

But one day, John's fervor caught up with him. As he was running, his skin suddenly felt very clammy and he became disoriented and dizzy. He felt nauseated, and his head pounded as if his running shoes were making tracks inside it.

John was suffering from heat exhaustion, a problem that occurs after long periods of exposure to extremely hot weather. Unlike heat-stroke, a life-threatening condition caused when our sweating system shuts down, heat exhaustion happens when we lose more water through sweat than we take in. It's a "drought" in the body.

The first thing to do for someone suffering from heat exhaustion is get him to the coolest place around. Place the victim on his back, raise his feet 8 to 12 inches and loosen his clothing. Give the person clear juice or water, provided he isn't vomiting. (If the person starts to vomit, stop giving fluids.) Apply cool, wet cloths, use a fan or move the person to an air-conditioned room. If the symptoms worsen or persist for more than an hour, get medical help.

But that's emergency care. It's better to prevent the problem in the first place. Keeping your body hydrated is the best way to avoid heat exhaustion. But not all liquids are created equal. Hanging out with a frosty beer or a gin and tonic is not your best bet for keeping cool. After a few sips of alcohol, you'll actually feel *warmer* because alcohol calories are burned quickly, raising your metabolic rate and your body temperature. Stick to cold water. It's absorbed into the body faster than warm water, cooling you down fast.

"Water and fruit juice are the best replacement fluids," says T.

Stephen Jones, M.D., a researcher at the government's Centers for Disease Control in Atlanta, Georgia. "But don't use thirst as a guide for how much to drink—it's inaccurate. Drink more than you're thirsty for."

With each drop of sweat, your body loses potassium and magnesium, two nutrients that are vital to the body's temperature-regulating mechanism. To replace these key nutrients, eat lots of foods rich in them. Fruits and fruit juices have lots of potassium. Other good sources for these nutrients are beans, spinach, potatoes, chicken, tuna and salmon.

Vitamin C also helps people resist the heat. Gold mine owners in South Africa found a daily supplement of 250 milligrams of vitamin C enabled most of the workers to acclimate to the intense heat in the mine shafts in half the usual time.

One nutrient you don't have to take steps to replace is salt. "It's not necessary to consume more salt in the summer," says George Jessup, Ph.D., a professor at Texas A&M University. "Most water supplies have higher salt levels than recommended, and the average American gets enough in foods." Forget about salt tablets, too. "Salt tablets are dangerous for people with heart disease or a disposition toward it," says George Poda, M.D., of Aiken, South Carolina, "And sometimes they make even healthy people sick."

Exercising until you drop from heat exhaustion is simply not virtuous. "Any exerciser working out in the first few weeks of summer heat can't expect to go out and do the amount of exercise he's accustomed to," says John Rockett, M.D., of Memphis, Tennessee. "Slow down the pace of biking, running, walking and other activities. Wear loose, light-colored clothing, and stay in shaded areas as much as possible. Head for places with grass, trees and water—asphalt is probably the worst exercise surface in the heat."

LEARN NOT TO BURN

Overdosing on sunlight not only ages the skin and causes wrinkles, it is also the single biggest factor in causing skin cancer, according to Allan L. Lorincz, M.D., professor and chief of dermatology at the University of Chicago.

This doesn't mean you have to stay away from the beach or forgo your favorite outdoor activities. But it does mean that you should invest in a good sunscreen. Sunscreens absorb, reflect or scatter the ultraviolet light of the sun, thus reducing the amount that will reach your skin.

Para-aminobenzoic acid (PABA), a B complex vitamin, is one of the most potent sunscreens you can obtain. It protects against the UVB wavelengths of the sun, the ultraviolet radiation that causes sunburn damage. At the same time, PABA permits UVA— the less dangerous tanning rays—to reach the skin.

Even better are PABA's derivatives, sometimes listed on labels as PABA esters or Padimate-O. These rarely stain clothing, as PABA can, and don't wash off as easily as PABA, yet they provide the same amount of sun protection. A word of caution: PABA and its derivatives can cause an allergic reaction in a small number of people. If you are one of them, try a sunscreen with different active ingredients. The Food and Drug Administration (FDA) lists 21 sunscreen ingredients that they consider to be safe and effective. Some of the most common include benzophenone, cinnamates and imidazol sulfonic acid compounds.

Carl S. Korn, M.D., assistant clinical professor of dermatology at the University of Southern California in Los Angeles, advises using a sun-blocking agent that has a Sun Protection Factor (SPF) of 15 or above. This number, listed on the label, indicates the amount of time you can stay out in the sun without burning. If you usually burn in 30 minutes, for example, a sunscreen with an SPF of 10 allows you to stay in the sun ten times longer without burning, or five hours. Sunscreening agents with an SPF under 15 filter out only some of the sun's harmful rays. Products with an SPF of 15 or above deflect the sun entirely.

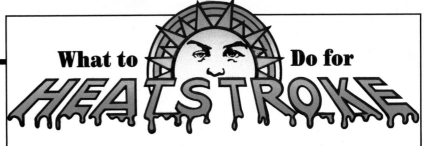

What to Do for HEATSTROKE

Long hours spent in scorching weather can bring on heatstroke, especially in elderly people and those who are diabetic, seriously overweight, dehydrated or suffering from sleep disorders. In heatstroke the brain mechanism that regulates body temperature quits working, and fevers can soar to 104° or more. This condition is life-threatening and merits immediate medical attention, preferably in a hospital emergency room. But minutes count, so until the medics come, here's what to do:

- Apply cold compresses to the victim's head. Then give him a sponge bath with warm water and alcohol. Make sure to bathe the underarms, groin and head, where heat is concentrated.
- Use an electric fan, a blow-dryer set to "cold" or a handmade fan to cool the victim.
- Keep the victim still in the shade or an air-conditioned room. If he's able to drink, give cold water. Don't give alcohol or drinks containing caffeine, since both are diuretics and would flush out precious fluids.
- Cover the person with a dry sheet and keep fanning him. If his temperature rises again, repeat these steps.

Apply a sunscreen liberally about 45 minutes to an hour before you head out into the sun so that the active ingredients have time to be absorbed. Claims on the labels notwithstanding, a good sweat or dip in the water will wash off the sun preparations, so reapply the lotion every two hours or after a swim.

Start by spending short amounts of time in the sun, and then increase them gradually. You can begin by spending 15 minutes sunbathing on the first day and add 5 minutes each day thereafter. Try to avoid sunbathing during the middle of the day. (The rays are strongest between 11 A.M. and 3 P.M.) Taking a dip in the water may cool you off, but it won't protect you from the sun's burning rays— ultraviolet rays travel right through water. This means you can still get a burn while swimming. And wearing a T-shirt in the water over your suit will do little or nothing to protect you. The water carries ultraviolet rays right through your clothing to your skin. The same holds true on land—you can get a burn through clothes soaked with water or perspiration. Keep a dry change of clothes handy.

Since sand reflects ultraviolet rays, you get a double dose of sun at the beach. Also, keep in mind that you can still burn on cloudy days. It's still quite possible to get from 60 to 80 percent of the amount of ultraviolet light you'd get on a clear day. And be especially careful at higher elevations, since the atmosphere is thinner and fewer harmful ultraviolet rays are filtered out. Staying in the shade won't necessarily protect you— this only reduces your sun exposure; it doesn't eliminate it.

COOLING REMEDIES

In case you've overdosed on sun, sizzling like a piece of poultry under a broiler, what can you do? Plenty. Home remedies for sunburn include everything from just plain cool water to cold tea or baking soda. Try some of these.

- Apply a generous dusting of talcum powder over the sore spots for quick relief.
- Soak in a tub of cool water. After the bath, apply cold, wet towels to the sore areas, rewetting the towels as they get warmed by the sunburn heat.
- Apply a thick paste made by mixing baking soda in water. This paste is an excellent first-aid dressing.
- Dilute vinegar with water and rub it on gently or add it to the bath water to alleviate pain.
- Apply some vitamin E ointment, or if you don't have the ointment, squeeze out the contents of several pierced vitamin E capsules and apply liberally. Vitamin E can reduce the temperature of the skin, relieve the pain and prevent blisters and peeling.
- Aloe vera is another terrific sunburn treatment. The gel or liquid from the aloe plant cools and moisturizes the skin and can prevent peeling.
- Apply some cold tea to sunburned areas. The tannic acid in the tea is an astringent and has been used by the Chinese as a pain reliever for years.

WHAT TO DO FOR FROSTBITE

Sunburn is skin damage at the hot end of the spectrum; frostbite is its opposite. Frostbite is actually a freezing of fluids in the skin and the underlying soft tissues. The small areas on the cheeks, toes, fingers, nose and ears, if exposed for a long period to extreme cold, are the most likely spots for frostbite. The signs of frostbite include red and painful skin, which then becomes white or grayish yellow and looks pale or glossy. Blisters may then appear. Often, another person will notice the symptoms of frostbite before the victim himself realizes he has it. Frostbite always requires professional medical attention.

This is a thermogram, taken by an infrared scanner. The scanner translates heat thrown off a body into a color spectrum. Areas of greatest heat loss show up white, yellow, red or pink. Surfaces that give off very little heat appear lavender, green, blue or black. This skier lost the most heat from his unprotected face and from his pelvic area, which normally generates a lot of body heat. His tight ski pants made heat loss even worse, since they restricted circulation, forced warm air out and let cold air in. The lesson: When you're out in the cold, layer up and avoid too-tight clothing.

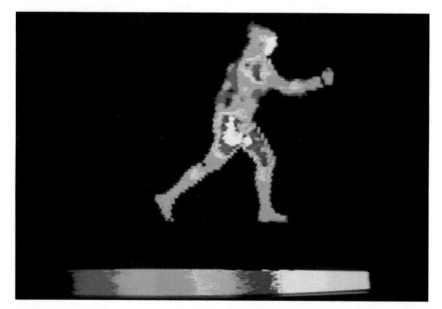

Layering: The Art of Keeping Toasty

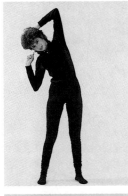

Three thin layers of clothing work better than 1 or 2 thick ones to shield you against winter's chills. That's because each layer traps air, which acts as insulation and retains body heat. The most effective layering serves 3 functions: vapor transmission (permitting perspiration to evaporate), insulation and protection.

The *vapor transmission layer*—the inner layer—should draw perspiration away from your body. The best materials for this job are polypropylene and olefin, both synthetics. Both are light, comfortable and better at removing moisture than cotton, which can feel cold and clammy when wet.

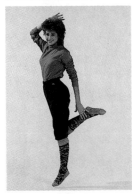

The *insulating layer*—a vest, shell, sweater or shirt—should be a lightweight but effective insulator so you can move around easily and generate your own heat. Fabrics such as Polar Guard, Hollofil II, Tex-Pro and Gore-Tex are some of the best materials for this layer. Pile and wool are also excellent since they retain warmth even when wet.

The *protective layer*—your parka, jacket, pullover or windbreaker—should shield you from wind and water, and protect your inner clothing layers. The best material for this outer layer is polytetrafluoroethylene (PTFE), a laminate that is waterproof but breathable, so your sweat will evaporate but snow, rain or moisture can't penetrate your clothes.

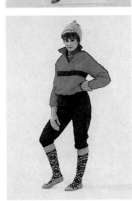

If someone has frostbite, the first thing you should do is protect the frostbitten area from further injury, then attempt to warm it. Cover the frozen area, making use of body heat; for instance, have the victim put his hands under his armpits. Get him to a warm area as quickly as possible, cover him with blankets and call for medical assistance.

You can also warm the frostbitten area by gradually immersing it in *warm* (never hot) water, about 100° to 104°F. If there is no water available, simply wrap the affected area in a blanket, sheet or other covering. Never rub the frozen area, since this action may cause gangrene, or tissue death. Give the victim something warm, like soup, to drink until you reach medical help. Encourage the person to move his toes and fingers after they are warmed. If possible, elevate frostbitten parts. Use dry, sterile gauze to separate frostbitten toes or fingers. And, if you do have to transport someone to a hospital or doctor's office for help, keep the frostbitten areas elevated and covered with a clean cloth.

It's also good to remember that once a foot, hand or cheek has become frostbitten, it is extremely vulnerable to future freezing. So cover up for safety, making sure you always protect your extremities with adequate headgear, footwear and gloves.

7

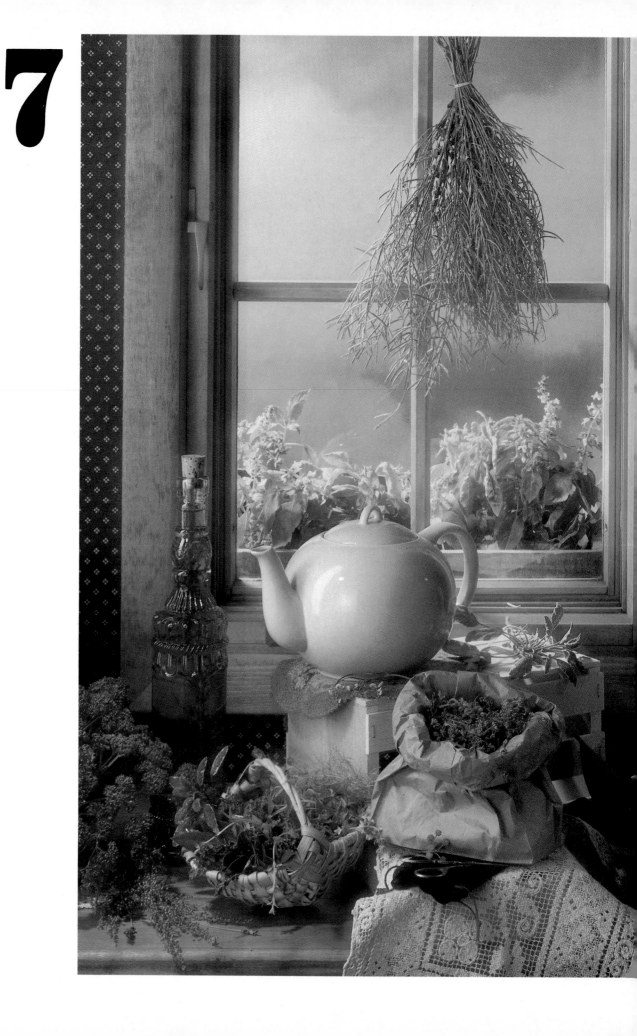

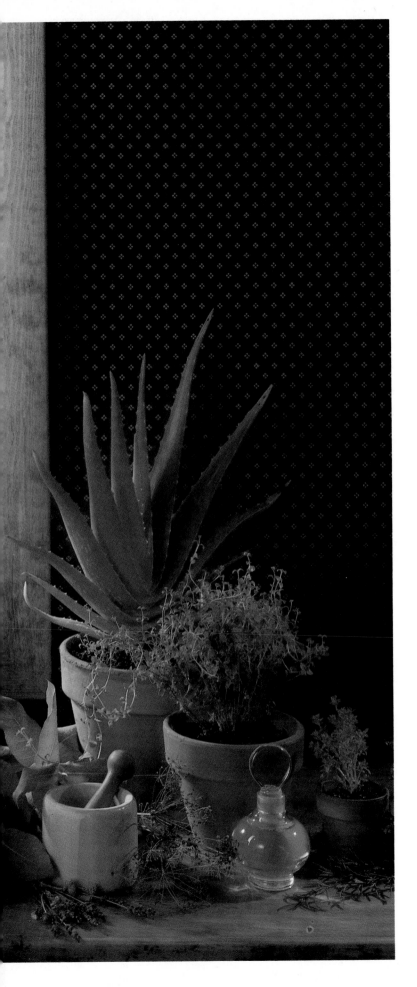

Folk Remedies: Another Look

Some withstand the test of time, others flunk. Here we sort the science from the lore.

Round about the cauldron go;
In the poison'd entrails throw,
. . . Fillet of a fenny snake.
In the cauldron boil and bake;
Eye of newt and toe of frog,
Wool of bat and tongue of dog. . .

For most people, folk remedies are about as scientific as this incanted concoction of *Macbeth's* witches. Many of the herbal remedies and healing practices that predated modern medicine have gone the way of "eye of newt," most with good reason. Much folk medicine was folk quackery—at best, worthless; at worst, lethal.

Take, for instance, pennyroyal, long an herbalist's cure for anything from stomach gas to unwanted pregnancy. The oil of this herb has been found to cause severe liver damage, even in small doses. That soothing cup of comfrey tea? It causes liver cancer in lab animals. (Now we're not saying that a few cups of pennyroyal or comfrey tea will give you cancer. But, in huge doses, these teas *did* harm experimental animals.)

But that doesn't mean all traditional remedies deserve the same fate.

Garlic, once used to ward off vampires, is now being tested in India for its ability to ward off cardiovascular disease. And scientists at several U.S. universities determined that activated charcoal can be as effective a poison antidote as legend says it is.

Some old-time remedies have even found their way to the pharmacist's shelf. An estimated 25 percent of all prescriptions dispensed today contain active ingredients from plants known in medical folklore.

Lovely...But Dangerous

Your grandmother may have shoved a cup of sassafrass tea at you for every little ache and pain. Your local herbalist may still prescribe a brew of blue cohosh for "female troubles." And in the back of your mind, you know that foxglove is good for the heart. But beware! This particular bouquet of herbs and flowers is nothing more than pretty poison—and in most cases, as therapeutic as a sugar pill. The ones that do have value, like foxglove, are safe only under the best of circumstances: When processed in a laboratory and prescribed in the correct dosage by a doctor.

Mistletoe

Kiss under it, but don't make tea from it. It contains substances that caused weakening of the heartbeat and a drop in blood pressure in test animals.

Blue Cohosh

This American Indian remedy has been used traditionally for "female conditions." The Indians called it squaw root. Avoid it for any condition. It can seriously damage the heart muscle.

Goldenseal

An old Indian remedy, goldenseal became the darling of patent medicine hucksters. But you'd need a near-toxic dose of this bitter tonic for the drug to be of only dubious therapeutic value.

Foxglove

The old herbalists used it for dropsy (edema). Today, doctors use foxglove—known as digitalis—to treat congestive heart failure. But it's no home remedy. Every part of the plant is poisonous. Children are often made ill just by sucking on the flowers. A mere 6 ounces will kill an ox.

Coltsfoot

Its Latin name comes from a word meaning "cough." For centuries, coltsfoot was a popular remedy for coughs and bronchial congestion. But recently, Japanese scientists found the plant's dried flowers caused liver tumors in rats. The rest of the plant appears to be carcinogenic as well.

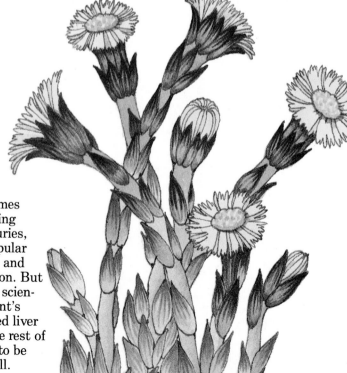

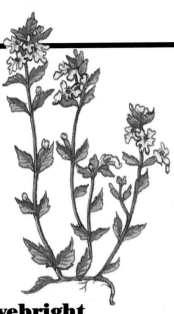

Daffodil

If you see a host of golden daffodils, admire, but don't eat them. Ingested in even small amounts, they cause nausea, vomiting, diarrhea, trembling and convulsions. Leaves and bulbs can also cause dermatitis in some sensitive people.

Eyebright

A fabled eye remedy because of its resemblance to bloodshot eyes, this ancient herb has no therapeutic value. To use it is to risk serious eye infection.

Rue

Once used to ward off the plague, this odoriferous shrub can relieve cramps. But the same antispasmodic agent can blister the skin if used in a poultice. It can also cause gastric upset when swallowed.

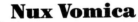

Nux Vomica

It does aid appetite and digestion. It's also an effective circulatory and respiratory stimulant. But its more common names—poison nut and strychnine—give more than a clue to its dangers. For a dose of nux vomica to be therapeutic, it has to come very close to being toxic, too.

Juniper

You may know the flavor. Juniper berries are used in sauerkraut, its oil in gin. Juniper is also an effective diuretic. But in excessive doses it can produce severe kidney irritation. It should be avoided by those with kidney disease.

Sassafrass

Once used to flavor root beer, sassafrass contains a cancer-causing agent called safrole. One cup of tea can contain up to 4 times the amount considered hazardous if taken on a regular basis.

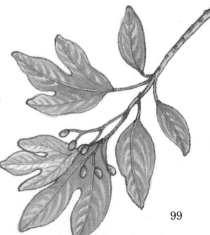

Remedies That Work

Science has shown many traditional herbal remedies to be useless—or dangerous. But some old folk medicines actually work.

Light, flowery *camomile* contains substances that will calm the stomach and protect against peptic ulcers. It has anti-bacterial properties, too.

Don't drink *comfrey* tea, but do use the root as a poultice. It contains allantoin, which stimulates cell growth to help wounds heal faster.

Uva ursi—that's *bearberry*—can be an effective urinary antiseptic if taken in correct dosages.

Cats love *catnip,* and so do insomniacs. Taken as a tea, it acts as a mild sedative.

99

Herbalists Today___

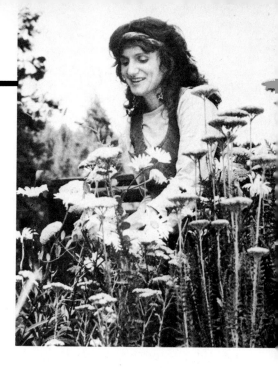

As a child, Leslie Kaslof couldn't tell sassafrass from sarsaparilla. In his Brooklyn neighborhood, nature was an even row of trees anchored by concrete. He found herbalism—and a way of life—during a chance encounter in the woods of northern California. "I ran into a friend who was studying with an Indian medicine man," recalls Kaslof. "He told me he was identifying plants with medicinal properties. I said, 'Do you mean, take this plant and chew it and my headache will go away?' He said, 'No, that plant is good for sore throats. *That* plant's good for headaches.'

"I felt as if lightning struck. I suddenly realized you could go out in nature and find something to heal your body. I was in awe."

Kaslof soon began walking the woods himself, herb books in hand. Eventually, he set up a herb co-op in the San Francisco Bay area and established what may have been the country's first "herb bar" at a natural foods restaurant in Sausalito. At the same time, the former journalist was collecting and experimenting with herbal remedies, poring for hours over ancient *materia medicas* and formularies.

In the early 1970s, Kaslof drove through Mexico to British Honduras, exploring Central American herb bazaars and trading secrets with native medicine men and women. "I was like a kid in a candy store. The whole world opened up to me," he says.

Kaslof, in turn, has opened up the world to others. As well as being a healer, he is the author of several herb books and a widely used herb chart. Today, he is also executive director of the national training and certification program for the Dr. Edward Bach Healing Centre.

Kaslof discovered the Bach Flower Remedies a dozen years ago. Developed by a British doctor, the healing system relies on 38 flowers—most indigenous to Great Britain—picked and specially processed only at certain times of the day and during certain phases of the moon. Unlike many herbs and drugs, the flower remedies do not work in a direct pharmacological way, says Kaslof. Rather, they act as catalysts to encourage the body to produce its own healing agents.

"Dr. Bach said that disease was basically beneficent because it allows us access to resources we'd never touch otherwise—our own healing capacity," Kaslof explains.

The Bach Flower Remedies are said to soothe the psyche as well as the body, and Kaslof believes that in the next decade, this largely arcane healing system will help move medicine from its pharmacological base to a truly holistic one that recognizes that integrity of body and soul. "This," he says, "is future medicine."

___

One of Rosemary Gladstar's earliest memories is of her Armenian grandmother's herbal foot baths. "She gave them to me and my family as a form of relaxation," she recalls. "She would take all her grandchildren to help her pick

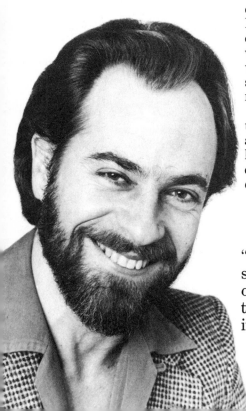

"I felt as if lightning struck. I suddenly realized you could go out in nature and find something to heal your body. I was in awe."

Leslie Kaslof

chickweed, purslane and dock. Herbal healing was part of our lives. My parents had five kids and they never took us to the doctor. We never thought that was odd. It was just the way it was."

Rosemary Gladstar runs an herb store in the Russian River area of California's Sonoma County, conducts holistic healing retreats and herbal caravans to the Baja Peninsula, Death Valley and into the Alaskan hills. She also finds time to operate a free herbal clinic at her home.

Though herbalism may have come naturally to her, Rosemary Gladstar sowed more than a few wild oats before she began collecting them. She hiked and lived alone in rustic cabins and pitched tents in the Canadian Rockies and the Trinity Alps of California and fulfilled a lifelong dream to ride horseback into the hills—which she did with her two-year-old son, Jason, strapped to the back of a palomino.

She had earned the money for the horses by working in an herb store and after the 4½-month trip, opened the shop she operates today. "We have 300 different herbs at least," she says.

She prefers to collect the herbs herself and use the ones indigenous to her northern California home. "It follows the idea of the relationship between illness and the environment," she says. "What's around you causes it; therefore, what's around you can heal."

For several years, Rosemary worked closely with a physician. As far as she is concerned, it was too closely. "You need to find where your own power is," she says, "and sitting in a doctor's office is not where I have the most joy."

But it was more than her own happiness that concerned her. The herbalist, she says, draws the power to heal from the "forces of life"; the physician draws it from the forces of science. When the twain meet, they don't always mingle well.

Though herbalism has gained in legitimacy, Rosemary says she fears the day it becomes institutionalized. "Once you become legitimate, who sets the standards? Not herbalists, but the Food and Drug Administration, which has no understanding of herbology. Then," she says, "we really will have lost something."

When Nan Koehler took one of her first classes in herbal medicine, she noticed that her instructor made more than a few mistakes when identifying healing plants. But then, Nan had an advantage—a master's degree in botany from the University of Chicago.

"Later, I took one class with herbalist Jeanne Rose and she had me take students on little herb walks during class," says Nan, a midwife and mother of five in California. "I knew all the plants, but at school they don't teach you how to do anything with them."

And Nan wanted to know. It was in her background. Her mother had a doctorate in biochemistry and treated her children's sniffles and fevers with herb teas. Her grandmother collected and painted wild flowers.

Nan read voraciously and took more classes (in one of which she met her future husband, an obstetrician). "We later worked together. He was really interested in learning about remedies and using them in his practice," she says. "But he was so severely criticized by his peers he had to back off from that."

Nan is used to that reaction from the medical community, which regards herbal medicine as something akin to shamanism. "They think it's some kind of mysterious witchcraft," she laughs. "It's really simple and scientific. I'm the most scientific person I know!"

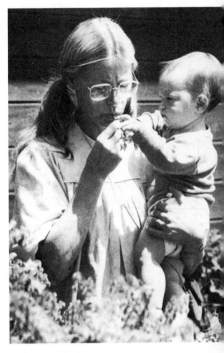

EDITOR'S NOTE: Doctors and herbalists may disagree on the effectiveness of herbal remedies to treat various conditions. Herbal remedies are not cure-alls and may not be effective for you. You should seek competent medical assistance for any condition that recurs or fails to respond to treatment.

Food Remedies

Mineral Water: Healthy or Not?

Even though it tastes good (or at least not bad), is mineral water really good for you, as so many ads imply?

Well, it doesn't have any calories, which is certainly an advantage over soda or alcohol. But it can contain large amounts of sodium, a negative for folks who already have high blood pressure. Yet for people who want to *prevent* that problem, mineral water contains small amounts of calcium, potassium and magnesium, minerals that may help keep the lid on blood pressure.

But the main advantage of bottled water—whether it's from a spring or a well or in distilled form—is its reasonable purity: It has none of the chemical pollutants that can make public water such a questionable soup.

When your mother cautioned you to "drink your milk, it will give you strong bones" and "eat your carrots, they're good for your eyes," she was intuitively practicing preventive medicine. It didn't mean much to you then, but when you grew up you learned that milk is full of calcium that does indeed build strong bones, and carrots are rich in vitamin A, so necessary to night vision.

Your mother was right on target with her advice, just as Hippocrates was 2,300 years ago when he counseled, "Let food be your medicine and medicine be your food."

We know that eating the right foods—like milk and carrots—can keep us healthy. But there also are certain foods that heal us when we're not. Anyone who has ever sipped a comforting cup of warm milk to lull himself to sleep or drunk tart cranberry juice to relieve a urinary tract infection knows the age-old wisdom of these "edible cures."

And along with the wisdom, there's solid research. That glass of warm milk contains tryptophan, an essential amino acid that has been shown in laboratory tests to induce drowsiness and promote a deeper, more restful sleep. Cranberry juice contains an antibacterial agent that can relieve the symptoms of chronic urinary tract infections.

You may have given your grandmother a condescending smile when she recommended a dose of bran for "what ails you." Today, scientists know that bran, the coarse outer hull of the grain of wheat, acts like a sponge in the gastrointestinal tract, absorbing water and waste and expelling it quickly. That makes it a safe, natural preventive measure for constipation and, surprisingly, for cancer. Researchers believe that the dietary fiber in bran dilutes toxins, like those that cause cancer, and whisks them out of the body before they can do any harm. Also, studies of populations whose diets were high in fiber showed they had fewer diseases of the colon and suffered less from heart disease, diabetes, hiatal hernia and appendicitis. So score one for Granny.

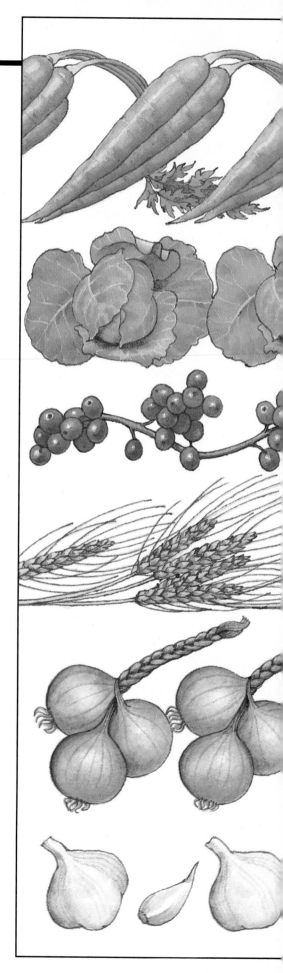

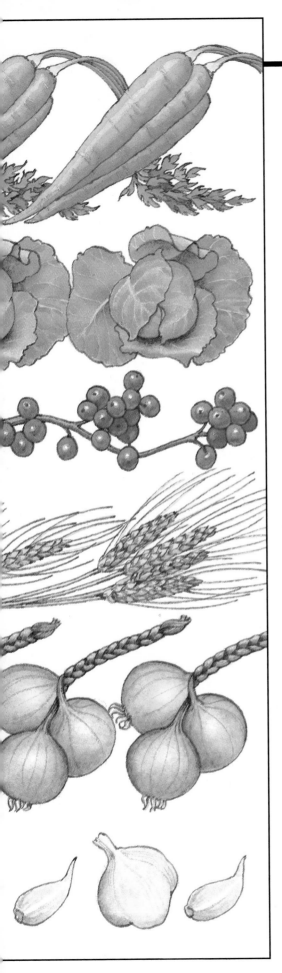

Ulcer trouble? Put down the milk and reach into the vegetable crisper for cabbage. A team of doctors at University College Hospital Medical School in London tested a wide variety of foods on rats to determine which ones protected against ulcers. The clear winner was raw cabbage, which, rather than protecting the stomach wall directly, reduced the amount of potentially harmful natural stomach acids needed for digestion. In the writings of Pliny, we learn there was an entire book, now lost, on the "cabbage therapy" of ancient Greece, where the vegetable was used for, among other things, hangovers.

If you have a bottle of apple cider vinegar in your pantry, along with a jar of honey, you can whip up a cold remedy faster than you can say "Gesundheit." Like over-the-counter cold syrups, yours will contain an irritant to break up mucus—the vinegar—and an ingredient to soothe the throat—honey. (You can substitute lemon juice for vinegar if you prefer its flavor.)

Folk healers swear by onions and garlic, and doctors are beginning to sing their praises, too.

Garlic contains a substance called alliin, which, when ground, becomes allicin, a powerful antibacterial agent. This property makes garlic useful in warding off a variety of common maladies.

Garlic is an expectorant that can help clear up colds, coughs, sore throats and even sinus infections. It is said to relieve stomach and intestinal ailments, including diarrhea and colic in infants. It has even been reported to kill warts. Garlic should be taken orally for all of these ailments; it's available in capsule form to avoid bad breath.

Onions are also something of a wonder. Poultices of onions are said to heal minor bruises and boils. Another home remedy uses raw onions applied to a sting to take down swelling and alleviate some discomfort. Eating onions can even protect against heart disease by reducing the tendency of the blood to clot.

Spices of Life

Cinnamon
The aromatic oil from this common culinary spice acts both as a digestive aid and as an antiseptic.

Cardamom
The volatile oil distilled from the dried, ripe seed of this spice can help relieve gas.

Cloves
You can use them whole to stud a ham—or ease an aching tooth with their oil. Oil of cloves is also an antiseptic.

Anise
Frequently mistaken for licorice, anise is a popular flavoring agent. It's also a diuretic and an expectorant, good for colds. (Don't use anise oil, though; it can be toxic in small doses.)

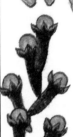

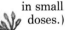

Ginger
Not only a cure for motion sickness (see "Ginger Root for the Road" on page 84), ginger is also a safe and effective soother for any stomach upset.

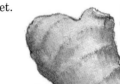

Healing the Skin

There are probably more folk remedies for the skin than for any other organ. And that's not really a surprise; it is, after all, the envelope in which we live. Skin, more than any other part of the human body, suffers the slings and arrows of outrageous living. We can damage it, even accelerate the aging process, if we fail to protect ourselves against the ravages of excessive exposure to the elements. Then, too, the skin's pores absorb the same environmental pollutants we breathe. Poor nutrition, lack of exercise, even stress can show first in our complexion.

SKIN CELL REGENERATORS

The aloe plant has played a prominent role in the folk healer's pharmacopoeia for 18 centuries. It is still the skin's best friend. You can help heal minor burns or abrasions simply by snapping off a leaf and squeezing the cool juice on the affected area. Aloe also conditions the skin and reportedly eases the symptoms of poison ivy. Chemically it's a real healer. Studies show that aloe promotes the growth of human cells. In fact, a group of physicians at a Chicago burn center used the mucilagenous juice of the aloe plant, along with aspirin, to heal 43 of 44 frostbite victims without major tissue loss.

"These results are startling; a much greater amount of tissue loss is usually associated with frostbite injuries," says one of those physicians, Martin Robson, M.D., professor of surgery at the Pritzker School of Medicine at the University of Chicago.

Aloe—Use It Fresh

When it comes to aloe vera, you're better off growing your own. Wendell Winters, Ph.D., of the University of Texas Health Science Center, tested store-bought aloe on human cell cultures and found it didn't work as well as fresh extract. He believes that commercial preparations contain chemicals that actually inactivate the healing properties of the plant extract. Your best bet is to keep an aloe plant handy so you can snip off a leaf and squeeze out the healing gel as needed.

Comfrey root is another old-fashioned remedy that promotes healing cell growth. Its active ingredient is allantoin, used in many commercial skin care products today. Comfrey root makes an excellent poultice for sunburn, wounds, boils, bruises or skin ulcers. (See "How to Prepare a Poultice" on page 106.)

KITCHEN-COUNTER CURES

You probably have some first-rate skin healers right in your kitchen. The same substance that sparks up your salad dressings is a tried-and-true skin soother as well: apple cider vinegar. It can reduce the swelling of an insect bite, ease the sting of sunburn and relieve rashes and athlete's foot. Since bacteria thrive in alkaline environments, ½ cup of vinegar added to a shallow bath can acidify the water to help clear up many stubborn vaginal infections by discouraging bacterial growth.

According to Robert M. Taylor, M.D., author of *Dr. Taylor's Self-Help Medical Guide,* a poultice made of grated raw potatoes applied repeatedly to small lacerations will help prevent infection and encourage healing. Cabbage juice or boiled cabbage leaves will achieve the same end, the physician says. Dr. Taylor prescribes the spud for poison ivy, too.

ITCH TREATMENTS FROM SCRATCH

Plagued by itching? Naturopathic physician Stan Malstrom, M.D., uses a tea of yellow dock and plantain to treat itches. But you don't drink it—you apply it to the itchy area instead. Packs of clay, comfrey, chickweed and yellow dock are also in Dr. Malstrom's black bag of treatments for itchy skin. If it's a mosquito bite that's driving you crazy and you don't have any herbs handy, he suggests placing a piece of adhesive tape over the bite to reduce the itching.

Prickly heat, or heat rash, that other plague of hot summer nights, is an inflammation of the sweat glands that raises tiny red bumps on the skin, often where belts or collars bind. Your mother's old treatment—a dusting of talc—will usually work, as will a colloidal oatmeal bath and your trusty old friend, the aloe plant. (See "Vitamin C and Prickly Heat" on page 92 for another cure.)

HEALING WITH VITAMIN E

One popular home remedy that has the support of some pretty impressive evidence from the laboratory is vitamin E. As every mother, schoolteacher and camp counselor knows, it will hasten the healing of a skinned knee, scratched shin or scraped elbow.

Researchers at the Harvard Dental School used vitamin E in a study of gum wounds and discovered—much to their surprise—that it made wounds heal much faster.

David C. Salter, Ph.D., associate director of the Xienta Institute for Skin Research in Bernville, Pennsylvania, rubbed some vitamin E on the back of mice he subjected to a dose of ultraviolet light, to simulate the burning rays of the sun. His discovery? Vitamin E acts as an effective sunscreen, reducing the amount of light reaching the skin and cutting down the cell damage that's part of sunburn.

Dr. Salter and his associates also discovered another use for E: as an anti-inflammatory. They rubbed a cream containing vitamin E into the skin of test subjects and electronically measured changes in the blood flow through the capillaries. (The major characteristic of inflamed skin is leaking of fluid from capillaries, the tiniest blood vessels, into the tissue.) The result was reduced flow, caused, Dr. Salter theorizes, by a narrowing of the capillaries, an action brought about by the vitamin E. "It's clear," he says, "that if you apply vitamin E topically when the skin is damaged, it will help to reduce the whole inflammatory process."

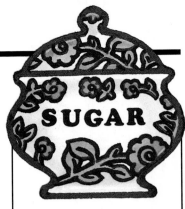

The Healing Power of Sugar

A 73-year-old woman whose fingertip was amputated when slammed in a car door recovered completely in 4 weeks with no scarring, thanks to an old-time remedy: sugar. The man who rediscovered the remedy—Richard Knutson, M.D., of Greenville, Mississippi—has treated more than 2,000 wounds, burns and skin ulcers with table sugar and iodine.

Here's how to use Dr. Knutson's cure: Mix 4 parts sugar to 1 part Betadine ointment (available at drugstores) and apply the mixture to cuts that have stopped bleeding. (If a cut is still bleeding, sugar will make it bleed more.) Cover with gauze and repeat as needed.

Poultices and Plasters

A frantic mother reportedly used a poultice of plantain leaves to heal an ugly, glass-filled gash in her daughter's foot. Not only did the poultice soothe the wound, it drew a large sliver of glass from the little girl's foot.

The Bible tells us that the prophet Isaiah used a poultice of figs to cure King Hezekiah of a nearly fatal boil infection.

Clearly, you don't need a degree in pharmacy science to use a poultice, an ancient form of healing bandage.

A poultice is actually a warm, moist paste of herbs commonly used to treat inflammations, bites or other skin irritations. You can use powdered, crushed or boiled herbs in a poultice, mashing them into a paste with oatmeal, flour or another mushy grain. According to one expert, 2 ounces of herbs should be mixed with 20 ounces of paste.

You can apply a poultice directly to the skin—after touching the paste to be sure it's not hot enough to scald you—or you can apply it indirectly by placing the herbal concoction between two strips of a thin cloth like gauze.

California herbalist Nan Koehler sometimes crushes a fresh herb and places it directly on the skin, holding it there with a gauze wrap.

One of the best-known poultices is usually not called a poultice at all. It's a mustard plaster, used over the ages to relieve the congestion of a cold. In case your mother has lost her recipe, here's another: Make a paste of 1 part crushed mustard seeds and 4 parts flour mixed with warm water. One expert advises placing an egg in the mixture to keep it from burning. Place the plaster mixture in a cloth, apply it to the area of congestion and slide it around to break up the mucus. You may want to rub the area where the plaster is to be applied with olive oil so it slides without chafing.

Nan Koehler sometimes uses a "decoction" in her poultices. "This is the best way to apply comfrey to the breasts to relieve soreness from premenstrual swelling," says this herbalist-midwife.

To make a decoction, soak the

How to Prepare a Poultice

When making a poultice with fresh herbs, simply crush the herbs in a blender or a mortar and pestle, then mix with a small amount of hot water. (In the case of a tough root like dock, steam until soft enough to mash.) If you use dried herbs, they must be crushed, mixed with a suspending material such as bran or cornmeal, then moistened with hot water to form a paste.

To apply the poultice, test the paste to make sure it is not too hot, then place it between squares of gauze or other thin cloth and apply to the affected area.

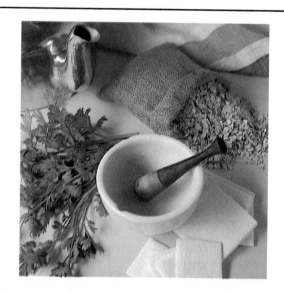

herb or root in cold water in a nonmetal container for about 10 minutes before heating to boiling. Simmer for 10 to 15 minutes and allow the mixture to steep for another 10 minutes, keeping the pot covered throughout the whole operation. Once you strain the liquid, you can either drink it as a tonic or use it in your poultice. (Comfrey should only be used externally.)

Herbs aren't the only poultice ingredient. Clay has been used since ancient times as a poultice and, believe it or not, as a therapeutic drink! To make a clay poultice, says Michael Abehsera, author of *The Healing Clay*, spread a layer of moist clay on a piece of cloth and apply it to a wound or inflammation so the clay comes into direct contact with the skin. (You can find clay at your local herbalist, health food store or riverbank!) Cover the poultice with a dry cloth, such as gauze, flannel or an Ace bandage. Abehsera also recommends using a cabbage leaf instead of cloth because the leaf will keep the clay moist longer. Generally,

he says, by the time the clay has dried and detached itself from the skin, it's done its job, although it can be reapplied.

Powdered charcoal is often used in poultices because of its remarkable ability to adsorb—bind to its surface—toxins and bacteria. To make a charcoal poultice, apply a ¼-inch layer of activated charcoal powder (available from drugstores) to the center of a thin, square cloth, like a handkerchief, and fold the four sides over the charcoal. Immerse the compress in warm water before applying it to the skin. Sometimes external heat from a hot water bottle or heating pad will enhance the effect.

To treat inflammation with a poultice, Dr. Malcolm Stuart, editor of *The Encyclopedia of Herbs and Herbalism*, recommends having these natural ingredients on hand: apple, carrot, coltsfoot, linseed, houseleek, oats, onion, parsley, comfrey and cucumber. Of course, any serious health problem should be treated by a physician.

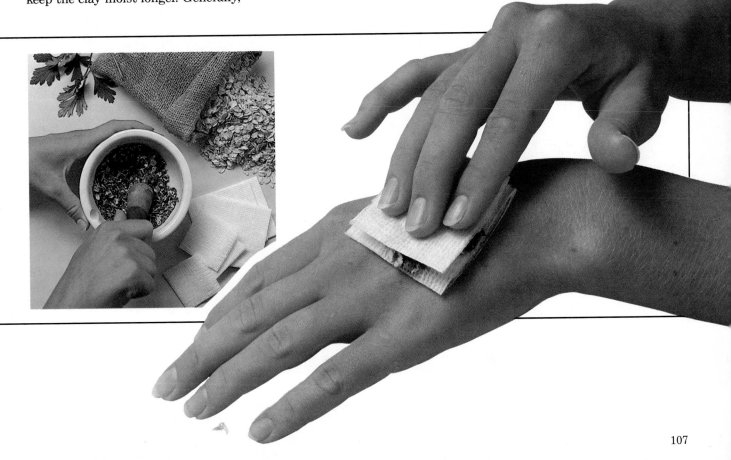

Folk Remedies from around the World

The English gave us the heart drug digitalis, synthesized from foxglove, a common plant with bell-shaped purple flowers. The South American Indians gave us both quinine, a treatment for malaria, and curare, used in surgery as a muscle relaxant. From China we get ephedrine, a drug used to treat asthma, hay fever and emphysema. For hundreds, even thousands of years before the discovery of the New World, healers from every corner of the globe had discovered uses for the bark of the trees and the flowers of the field. Fortunately, the efficacy of these cures made them worth handing down through the ages. Here are a few worth passing on.

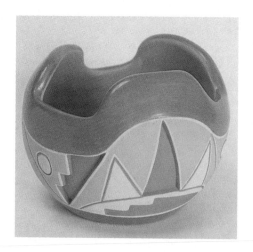

North America

The American Indians used slippery elm bark as a treatment for sore throats, diarrhea, toothaches, rheumatism and labor pains. Today, their wise old remedy is used only for sore throats. Slippery elm lozenges are a common, natural, over-the-counter throat soother.

Mexico

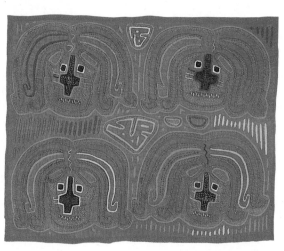

For centuries, natives of Mexico and other tropical regions where papaya grows have used it to treat intestinal worms, ulcers, eczema, warts and blemishes. Papaya's chief active ingredient, the enzyme papain, has been called a biological scalpel for its ability to digest dead tissues without harming live ones. Modern doctors have used papain to help heal a host of ills, including infected wounds and indigestion. The Food and Drug Administration has approved the use of papain injections to treat slipped disks.

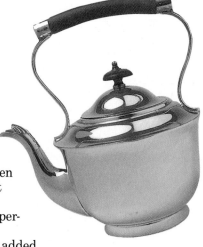

England

Since the late 1600s, the English have been using peppermint, a hybrid herb, to treat indigestion, gas and colic. According to pharmacognosist Varro Tyler, Ph.D., peppermint contains chemical substances that promote digestion, relieve gas and, as an added bonus, stimulate the appetite. Peppermint tastes good, too.

Japan

From the land of the rising sun comes shiatsu, a method of treating illness by pressing the fingers on certain pressure points. (Not all folk remedies are herbal!) One practitioner says the hand pressure "causes the springs of life to flow."

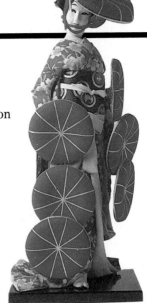

Arabia

Known from biblical times—it was a gift to the Christ child from the Wise Men—myrrh has been used as everything from incense to mouthwash— and still is. You'll find it in tooth powders and, as a tincture, myrrh is used to treat skin ulcers. When burned as an incense, it also repels mosquitos.

Italy

The most common use for hops is as a constituent for beer. Cultivated by the Romans, this wheatlike plant has a number of other, more therapeutic uses. It's a mild sedative, used alone or with other herbs to induce sleep. It's also a weak antibiotic.

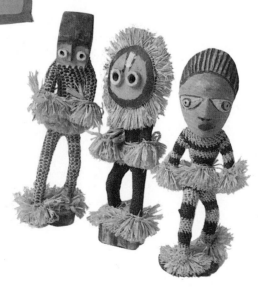

East Africa

Medicine men of East Africa use an herbal tea to ward off cholera—and it works. Scientists are now testing the antibiotic properties of the fruit of the *Maesa lanceolata* bush in the hope that someday it may be used widely as a cure for urinary tract infections and other bacterial diseases.

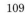

8

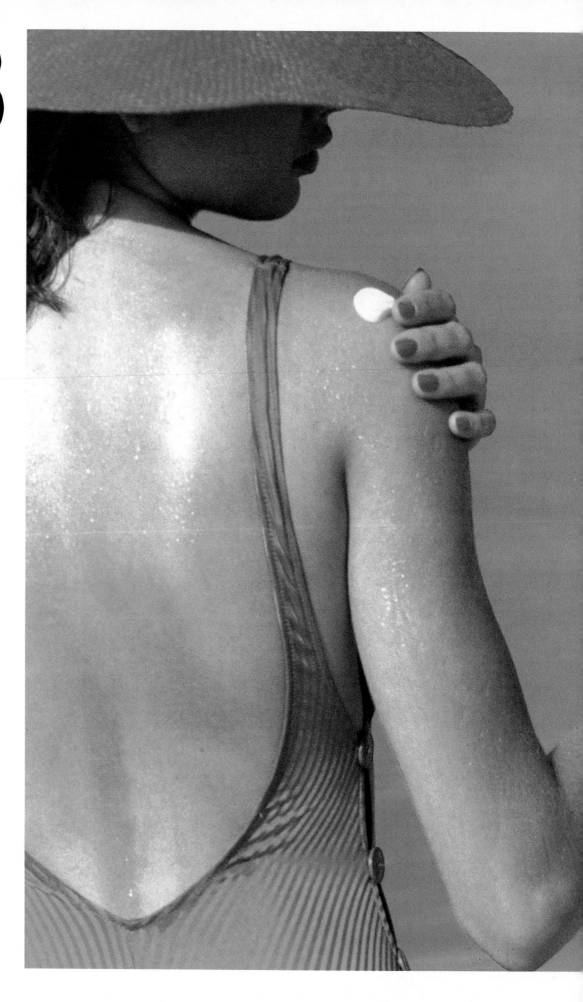

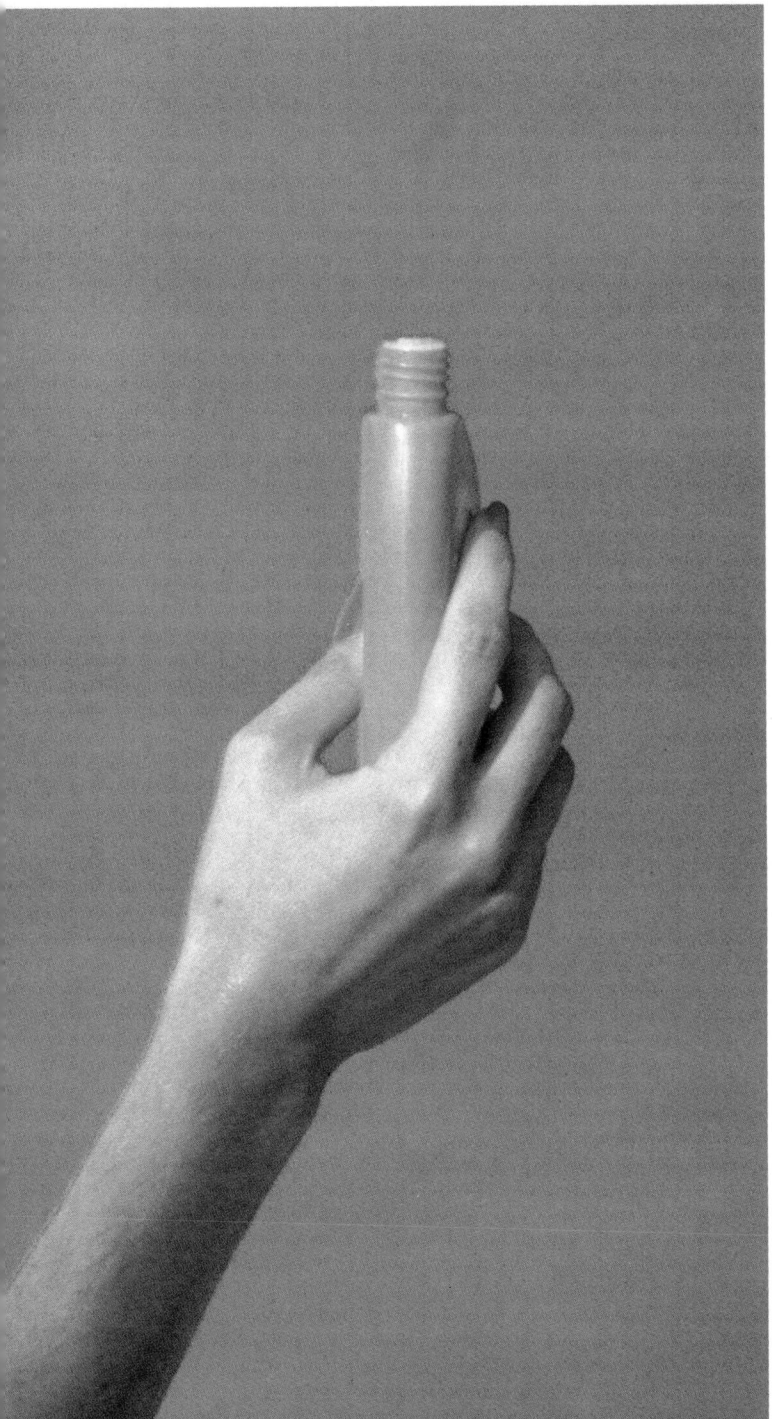

101 Health Hints

Fast, easy ways to make your life healthier—starting today!

1 Good suntan lotions these days have "Sun Protection Factor" numbers printed on their labels. These SPF numbers—ranging from 2 to 20—tell the burn-avoiding buyer how effective a sunscreen the product is; the higher the number, the better the screen. The accompanying chart shows you how to determine which SPF is best for you. As a general rule, multiply the SPF number on the label by the amount of sunning time it normally takes to turn your skin red the next day. For example, if an hour of sun usually makes you red, it will take 4 hours to get that red using a lotion with an SPF of 4, or 8 hours to get that crimson glow if the SPF is 8. To block out the sun entirely, an SPF of 15 or better ought to do the trick.

2 Here's a first-aid idea for pulls and sprains that need cold applied to them immediately to keep swelling down. Instead of fumbling with stubborn ice trays and ice cubes wrapped in dripping towels, use a bag or two of frozen vegetables—corn, peas or other small items. They're cold, they're handy, they're sturdy and they can easily be shaped to fit around whatever it is you've damaged.

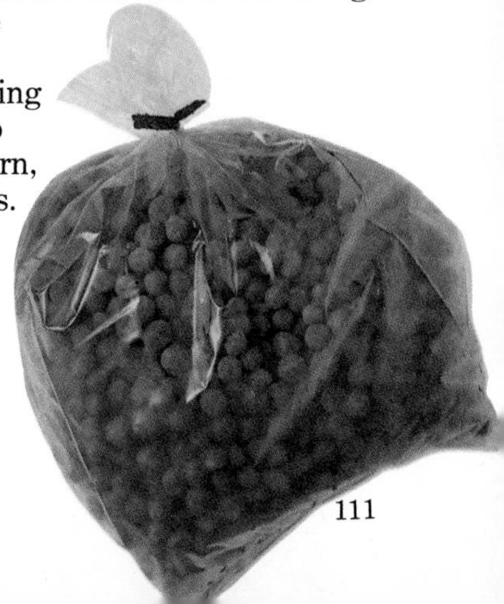

Sun Protection Factor

Type of Skin	SPF	Effect
Rarely or never burns or is deeply pigmented	2-3	Protects skin that's already tanned
Burns moderately, tans gradually and is fairly sensitive	4-5	Gives moderate sunburn protection yet still allows tanning
Burns easily, tans only a little and is sensitive	6-7	Gives high sunburn protection with only limited tanning
Burns easily, never tans and is sensitive	8-14	Gives excellent sunburn protection with very little or no tanning
Always burns easily, never tans, is sensitive and needs extra protection	15 or more	Blocks sun completely and protects extra-sensitive areas like bald spots, lips, ears and nose

3 On the other hand (or foot or knee), you could fill balloons with various amounts of water and freeze them. The best part of this is, you can make custom-fitting cold packs for any member of the family—and bright colors might help the kids get over their "booboo" trauma.

5 You can add years of energetic health to your life with a proper exercise regimen, but not by doing deep knee bends. In squatting positions your knees take a disproportionate amount of strain and your weight becomes unevenly distributed, forcing the knee ligaments and tendons to bear most of the load. Performing just one deep knee bend puts pressure on your knees equal to several times your body weight.

Here's a safe alternative: Pressing your back against a wall, bend your knees until your thighs are parallel to the floor, as if you're sitting on an imaginary chair. That way, your thigh and back muscles pick up the load.

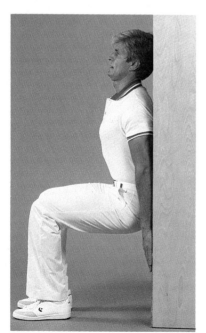

4

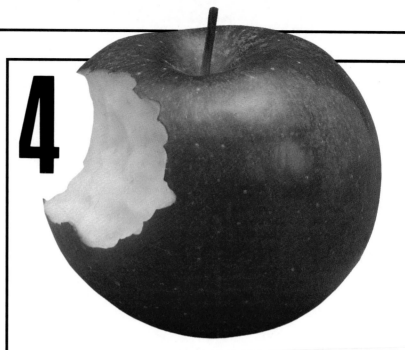

Those of us who can't seem to brush after every meal can stop decay-causing plaque from strip-mining our dental enamel by eating an apple after meals. Apples crunch among the teeth's spaces, dislodging the cavity creators and stimulating saliva flow to counteract plaque, says Elaine Parker, assistant professor of dental hygiene at the University of Maryland.

6

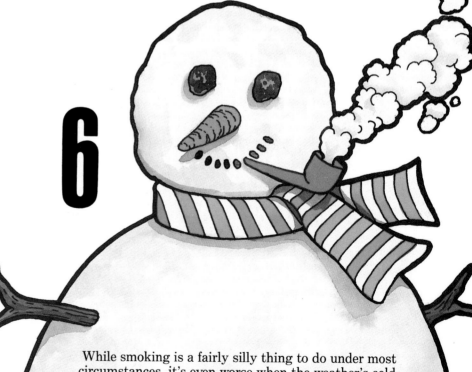

While smoking is a fairly silly thing to do under most circumstances, it's even worse when the weather's cold. Grabbing a smoke before you venture out into winter weather sets you up for frostbite by decreasing the flow of blood to your extremities—hands and feet, fingers and toes.

7

Sometimes a ring can't be pulled off an injury-swollen finger, setting up a vicious circle: The binding ring makes the finger hurt all the more. What to do?

Find a 3- or 4-foot length of string. Push a few inches of it between the finger and the ring and pull it through. If the finger's so swollen that the string doesn't pass through easily, use a matchstick, toothpick or some similar object to help push the string.

Then, wind what's left of the string in a tight spiral around the finger, starting at the edge of the ring and winding up toward the fingertip. Keep the circles close together.

Now, while keeping the string tight around the finger, grab onto the short end of the string (the part you passed between the ring and the finger), lift it so it's aimed toward the fingertip, and pull. The string will unwind, and the ring will follow until it's off the finger.

If the pain is simply too great to go fiddling with twisting twine, it's probably wise to see a medical professional.

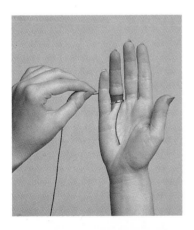

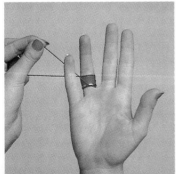

8

When looking for a good shampoo— especially when your hair's been damaged or bleached or permed—be sure to buy a kind that's "pH balanced." The pH number is an indication of how acid or alkaline a substance is. On a scale of 1 to 14, 1 is hydrochloric acid, way down on the acid end; 14 is the highest alkaline, bleach. Most soaps and shampoos are at 8 or 9, while water is a neutral 7. Trouble is, most hair is slightly acid, coming in at a pH of around 4.5 to 5.5. Seeking out and using a shampoo that's also between 4.5 and 5.5 pH undoes much damage to hair shafts, making them stronger, shinier and more manageable. Check shampoo labels for the pH.

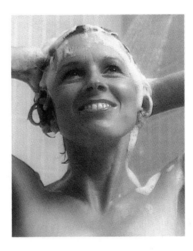

pH		
14	Alkaline	
13		Bleach
12		
11		
10		
9		Most soaps and
8		shampoos are pH 8 or 9
7	Neutral	Water
6		
5		Lemon juice is pH 5 or 6
4		Human hair is pH 4.5 to 5.5
3	Acid	
2		
1		Hydrochloric acid is pH 1

9

Chocolate may have been maligned as a dietary villain. A study at the University of Pennsylvania has exonerated the velvety brown stuff as a cause of acne. And figures from the U.S. Department of Agriculture show that a typical, plain, milk chocolate bar has 12 times more protein, 10 times more calcium, 10 times more phosphorus and 8 times more riboflavin than a medium-size apple.

But before you trash your apples and race for the candy store, consider that the chocolate bar also has 3 times as many calories, 28 times more fat and a crushing *40 times* more sodium than the apple.

Still, your occasional chocolate treats can be savored without guilt.

10

Don't buy too many new shoes the first time you're expecting. Many women's feet swell a half or a whole size after their first pregnancy. Why? Ligaments in both the pelvis and feet stretch when specific childbirth hormones order them to.

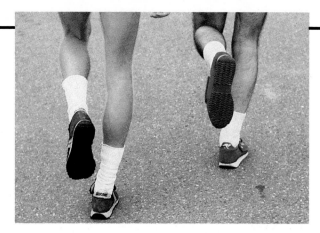

11

If you're often faced with some tough decisions, start jogging. After 20 people from a Midwestern farm community worked out 3 times a week for 6 months, they scored 70 percent better in a test of complex decision-making than before the exercise program. Simple 1-step decisions weren't affected by the program, and decision-making capacity is largely hereditary anyway, but regular invigorating exercise will make the most of your native ability to think clearly in a pinch.

12

Even during global energy crises, some of us never experience a shortage of natural gas. One flatulence sufferer decided to turn himself into a human guinea pig, isolating and testing more than 130 different foods to see which were major-league gas producers and which were safe, or at least safer.

In general, milk and wheat products were primary villains, probably because of the way bacteria in the colon react with carbohydrates. Here's how other foods rated:

Not Very Gassy. All meats, fowl, fish, nuts and eggs; lettuce, broccoli, tomatoes, asparagus, cantaloupe, grapes and berries; rice, corn chips, potato chips and popcorn.

Moderately Gassy. Pastries, potatoes, eggplant, citrus fruits, apples and bread.

Extremely Gassy. Milk products, onions, beans, celery, carrots, raisins, bananas, apricots, prune juice, pretzels, bagels, wheat germ and brussels sprouts.

13

What that new T-shirt does for you! You look so sexy, so clean, so *professional*, so—rubbed raw and sore. Wash that new shirt a few times before you run in it, because the material can chafe your upper torso, underarms, shoulders, neck and nipples. And it can't hurt to rub some petroleum jelly on any potential tender spots.

14

It's okay to dig into spicy eats, but just make sure they don't turn around and dig into you. Numerous cases have been reported where surgery was needed to extricate accidentally ingested bay leaves from where they'd pierced and gotten stuck in the intestinal walls. One preventive is to pick those bay leaves out of your pots, pans and trays before serving the meal. Another is to put the bay leaves in a small cheesecloth sack before dropping them in the saucepan.

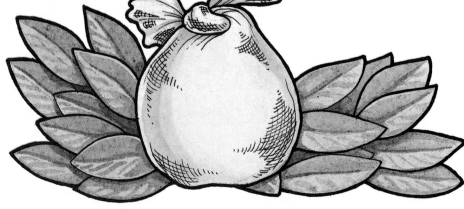

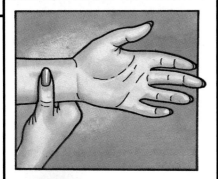

16 Have a rash you can't explain? Exercise a lot, too? Look to your equipment, at home or at the health club, as a possible culprit. Infection-causing bacteria are alive and well and ready to jog into your body, using exercise mats and other workout equipment as springboards. Regular disinfection should clear up the problem.

15 Try this if you're one of the 80 percent of pregnant women who suffer morning sickness: Press down on the acupressure points called "neikuans," which are located on the inner arm about three fingers' width from the crease at the wrist, toward the elbow. It's a technique that may work to either prevent the prenatal yuechs or get rid of them once they've come a-calling.

17 Pierced ears tingling with pain while jingling with jewelry are probably hypersensitive to some metals and alloys found in many earrings. To avoid this allergic reaction, buy earrings with stainless steel posts, or apply a coat of clear nail polish to act as an allergen barrier. Nail polish works on any other troublesome jewelry as well.

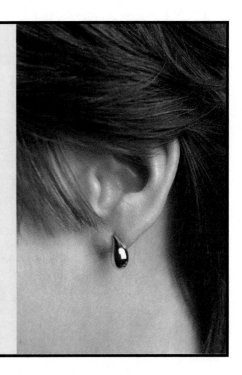

18 "Chinese restaurant syndrome"—a whole series of strange sensations, including warmth, stiffness, weakness in the limbs, headache, light-headedness, pressure and stomach upset—is a reaction to the monosodium glutamate (MSG) used liberally as a flavor enhancer in such establishments. At least one study suggests that the fault may lie not in our moo goo gai pan but in ourselves. Researchers say that the MSG sensitivity occurs because the eater has a vitamin B_6 deficiency. By taking 50 milligrams of B_6 daily, 8 out of 9 sensitive subjects lost their sensitivity.

19 When you're trying to jump off a weight-loss plateau, here's a trick to fool your body into shedding pounds faster: Raise your calorie intake every other day. A consistently low-calorie diet will slow your metabolism, but eating a few hundred extra calories every other day will help nudge it back into action.

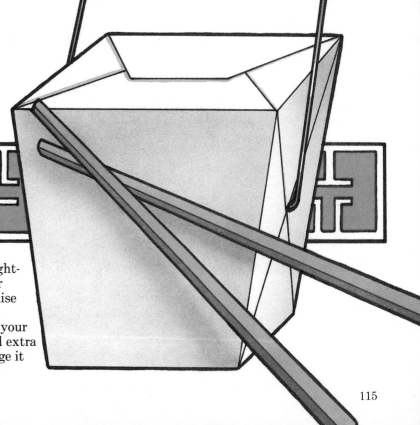

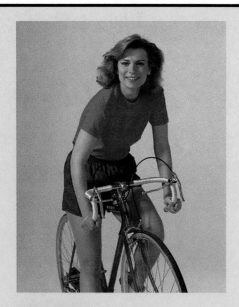

20 Timing. That's for comedians and mechanics, right? Now it seems it's essential for dieters, too. Studies have shown that aerobic exercise 1 hour after a meal helps burn off almost *twice* as many excess calories as exercise at any other time. So don't let an occasional calorie splurge get you down. Simply rest an hour after you eat (to avoid stomach pain), then get off your duff and work out.

21 The irresistible odors of fresh flowers or baking pies can act as tranquilizers. When a California psychologist tested the effects of certain aromas, including camphor and cinnamon, he found that the scents evoked joyful childhood memories among study participants. They also reported feeling surprisingly relaxed and refreshed.

So on days when you feel like a character in a Stephen King novel—tense enough to shatter glass at 20 yards—follow your nose to the nearest garden or bakery.

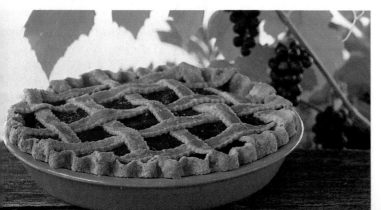

22 Poison ivy sufferers should be wary of certain booby-traps in their diet. Mangoes, for example, may be a hazard for the extremely sensitive; there's something just under the rind that'll do the same thing to you that poison ivy does. Also, the tiny pink peppercorn so popular in *nouvelle cuisine* is a member of the poison ivy family. These little peppers can hurt like all get-out if they get a chance to interact with your gastrointestinal tract. Avoid them at all costs.

23 There's a right way and a wrong way to blow your nose. Blowing so hard that you wreak havoc with your eardrums is, needless to say, the wrong way. The right way: Blow gently, keeping your mouth open. If both nostrils are stuffed up, blow them at the same time, not in alternating, heavy-duty honks.

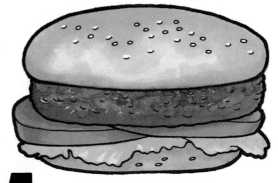

24 You may think that chicken is better than red meat for your heart and your waistline, but it ain't necessarily so—at least not in fast food restaurants. A hamburger with a bun can contain less fat than the fried chicken. If you do eat at fast food restaurants now and then, here are some decalorizing tips. (1) Eat low-fat foods for the day's other meals; (2) take off the chicken skin (where most of the fat and a lot of the calories are); and (3) try to stick to chicken that's been pressure deep-fat fried—decreasing cooking time means less contact with the fat and less nutrient loss. Of course, the best idea is to eat fried foods sparingly.

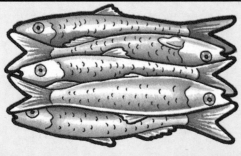

25

Maybe Great-grandma knew best. Scientists now agree that cod-liver oil *is* good for you. Certain fish livers and their extracts are high in eicosapentanoic acid (EPA), which seems to reduce cholesterol levels and act as a protective agent against cardiovascular disease. Two teaspoons a day of cod-liver oil provides about a gram of EPA—or about 10 times the present average intake level in some EPA-poor diets. Three ounces of herring or salmon, or liberal servings of sardines, anchovies and mackerel, are loaded with EPA, too.

26

If you're going crazy scratching the itch left on your epidermis by a mosquito— one of God's creatures that surely bites the hand that feeds it—just aim the warm, dry gusts of a hair dryer at the offending bump. That ought to soothe the spot and save your sanity for a while.

27

You wash your face, behind your ears, your feet and all those other places with soap. Now, researchers at Michigan State University think that perhaps you ought to wash your soap with soap, too. Long thought to be self-cleaning, a bar of soap can often harbor germs. In fact, some bacteria live on a cake of soap for up to 2 days, just waiting to be lathered into an open wound. The study showed that most healthy people will remain 99 and 44/100 percent pure and infection free, but those who want to slosh on the safe side ought to consider the far more germ-free liquid soaps that can be spritzed from hand pumps.

28

When your resolve starts to weaken on your new exercise regimen, pick some easy minimum goal. That way you'll placate your conscience; if you're feeling zippy, you'll exceed your own expectations. If that's *still* not enough to get you moving, get behind the most attractive swimmer, jogger or cyclist you can find. It's amazing how quickly your energy will return.

29

The cat has always been a symbol of sex and mystery and fertility. Today the symbol takes on new meaning because of a disease called toxoplasmosis, which is often carried by cats. This parasitic disease can infect pregnant women and cause birth defects, spontaneous abortion or stillbirth.

Cats pick up the parasite from infected birds or rodents and pass it through feces in the litter box or family garden. (The eggs may also be found in raw meat.) Toxoplasmosis is often asymptomatic but may make itself known in the form of swollen glands, fatigue, muscle pain, headache, sore throat, rash and fluctuating low fever. These symptoms usually fade quickly, except in pregnant women.

One of the two pharmaceutical treatments for toxoplasmosis also happens to cause birth defects, so the best course of action, if you plan to become pregnant, is prevention. Here's how:

- Avoid close contact with the cat throughout pregnancy.
- Keep the cat indoors so it can't hunt and eat mice and birds.
- Feed the cat only well-cooked meat or commercial cat food.
- Give the job of cleaning the litter box to another family member.
- Wear disposable gloves and wash your hands after working in gardens to which cats have access.
- Wash and/or cook homegrown foods that may have come in contact with cat feces in the garden.
- Wash your hands after touching uncooked meat.
- Cook meat at 150°F or higher.

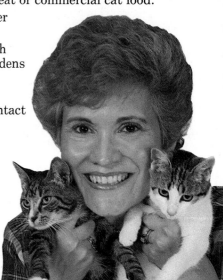

30

It's time to spread the truth about mayonnaise. Mayonnaise does not make foods spoil faster—it actually keeps them from spoiling! Studies have shown that the acidity of commercially prepared mayonnaise retards the growth of staphylococcus and salmonella bacteria in meat salads—even when the temperature is as high as 90°F. The more mayonnaise, in fact, the greater the protection. While mayo can't substitute for refrigeration, it's certainly safe for picnic meals.

31

Be sure to take off your rings when you wash your hands. If you don't, soap can get trapped between the ring and your skin and cause a bothersome rash. At least once a month, clean the inside of your rings with a brush, then soak them overnight in a solution of 1 pint of water and 1 table-spoon of ammonia. Rinse them thoroughly before donning them again.

32

Tossing and turning your first night in the country with no one but the raccoons for company? Or gritting your teeth at that nonstop roar outside your city friend's window? The problem could be that you're just not used to the change in nocturnal sounds.

Sleep researchers note it can take several nights to adjust to any nocturnal change, quieter *or* louder. Try playing a tape of the night noises you're used to drifting off to: A series of lulling records and cassettes from Atlantic Records called "Environments" features sounds of rain, a forest, the sea, summer cornfields, thunderstorms or even the heart. If you yearn for the soothing growl of buses, subways, car horns and clanging garbage cans, there's a cassette of city sounds called "Tin Pan Apple" available from Henri Bendel, 10 West 57th Street, New York, NY 10019.

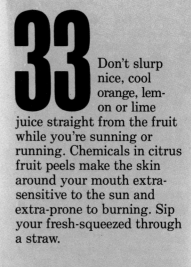

33

Don't slurp nice, cool orange, lemon or lime juice straight from the fruit while you're sunning or running. Chemicals in citrus fruit peels make the skin around your mouth extra-sensitive to the sun and extra-prone to burning. Sip your fresh-squeezed through a straw.

34

How can you take a nap that will leave you refreshed, rejuvenated and revitalized, not just groggier than before? Take a *short* one. Studies show that half-hour snoozes offer the same recharging powers as the 2-hour variety. Even a 10-minute catnap can do wonders. Timing helps, too. If you can, schedule your doze for about 2 P.M. That's when body rhythms naturally take a dip.

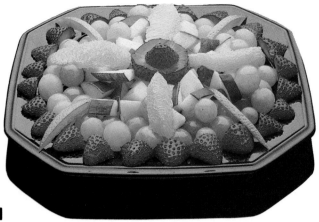

35

If hangover headaches are putting a damper on your holiday revels, reach for your fruit bowl. Research shows that fruit sugar can speed up your body's ability to burn alcohol. You can use it to head off your headache before the party or as a morning-after cure.

36

Bedridden with a common cold? Try using essential oils in your vaporizer for some relief. If you're running a fever and would like to cool down a bit, plunk a few drops of peppermint oil into the well of the machine. On the other hand, if chills are your problem add cinnamon oil, rosemary oil or basil oil to the vaporizer to warm you up. Vaporized eucalyptus oil is good for congestion.

38

If the log doesn't work, try dialing 212-772-7800. That's the telephone number for a 24-hour-a-day taped message by a New York City psychiatrist who will talk you to sleep. (Don't they all?) On the 8-minute tape, he gives you advice on attaining a relaxing position and speaks slower and s-l-o-w-e-r, and becomes boring and even more boring and repetitive and s-l-o-w-e-r, and you may soon . . . find yourself . . . dozing off . . . and . . . oops, dozed off ourselves for a second, just thinking about it. It works. But one warning: Be sure to hang up before you pack it in, or your phone bill could provide you with a rude awakening.

37

Sleepless nights don't just happen. There are reasons—and remedies. A good way to find both is to keep a record of your sleep, the theory being that you ought to keep a log if you want to sleep like one.

The point of the sleep log is to compare activities of the day to the quality and quantity of your snoozing. Over a 2-week period, a log can turn up all sorts of overlooked daily killers of sleep, and by seeing what these bogeymen are, you can put them—and yourself—to rest.

For each of the 14 days, make notations concerning:

- What time you go to bed
- What time you wake up
- About how long it takes you to fall asleep
- How long your night's sleep is
- How you feel in the morning
- What you eat
- What you drink
- What medications you take
- What activities you do in the evening before you go to bed
  - What kind and the amount of exercise you get during the day
    - How much coffee, tea, hot chocolate or cola you have from noon on (the caffeine in them might be keeping you up)
    - If you take any naps

    Look for common threads and patterns. Certain foods might make you toss and turn; so could not enough or too much exercise or a midday nap that leaves you too wide awake at day's end.

39

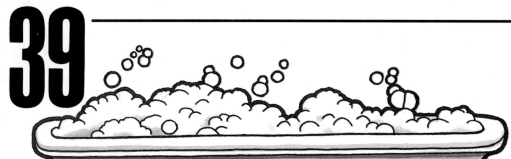

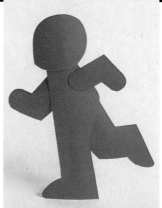

Our American zeal for cleanliness may help destroy our skin. As we age, our skin's production of oil slows down, and excessive washing makes it itchy and dry. Washing your underarms and crotch is enough to prevent odor, but if you are absolutely addicted to a daily bath or shower, use a moisturizer before you towel yourself dry, or squeeze bath oil into the tub.

40

Your friendly neighborhood pharmacist might be the most underrated health professional around. Pharmacy schools have started reemphasizing the importance of drug interactions, and new pharmacies have been designed with separate areas where you can confer with the pharmacist in private.

Though pharmacists aren't trained to diagnose, they can keep a watchful eye on potentially dangerous drug combinations that specialists working separately have advised you to take. If your condition isn't serious and you can adequately describe your symptoms, your druggist might also be able to recommend appropriate products.

41

The safe way to go when you jog daily along a busy road is to face the direction of oncoming traffic, so nobody with a multi-ton vehicle can sneak up on you. Just make sure you vary your route. If you run on the same side of the road every day, you invite "downside leg syndrome," the result of the approximately 14-degree slope for drainage built into many highway shoulders. The effects, including muscle atrophy, stress fractures and knock-knees, are the same as if one of your legs were shorter than the other.

42

If you wear gloves to avoid dishpan hands, use plastic gloves, not the rubber kind, says Stephen M. Schleicher, M.D.—rubber often causes hand dermatitis. Other tips: Don't wear the gloves for more than 15 to 20 minutes at a time; remove the gloves immediately if any water gets in; turn the gloves inside out and rinse them under hot water a few times a week and sprinkle them with talc to ensure dryness or wear cotton gloves under the plastic ones.

43

Do you get that irritating, gurgly and sometimes painful swimmer's ear when you hop out of the pool? And no matter how much shaking and pounding you do, it won't go away? Try putting a drop or two of rubbing alcohol into that waterlogged ear. It helps dry up excess moisture and keeps the ear canal clean. It's a mild antiseptic, too.

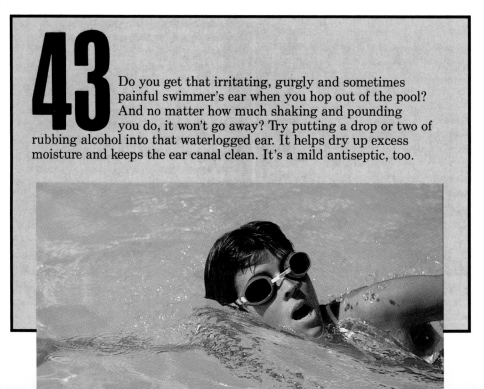

44 Accidents happen, and teeth have a way of parting company with the gums and ending up in the palm of a hand. Knowledgeable folks know that if the person can be transported to a dentist pronto, the tooth can likely be reimplanted and, with any luck, saved.

A dental researcher at the University of Florida has discovered that if the knocked-out tooth is quickly dropped in a glass of milk, the chances of its successful return to the living are greatly enhanced, as long as the trip to the dentist is a speedy one.

45 Got heartburn so bad you want a fire extinguisher? Try the old tried-and-true flame putter-outer—water. The best heartburn remedies are those that reduce the chance of bile or stomach acid backing up and searing the tender esophagus. By drinking a glass of cold water, you wash the acid off the esophagus and send it gushing back to the stomach where it belongs.

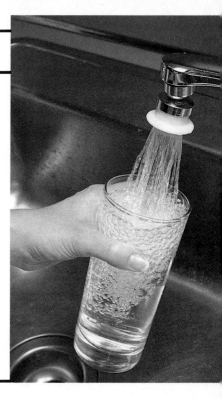

46 If you're working hard to unload some extra poundage, here's a simple formula to figure out how many calories are in the wine you drink: Find the percentage of alcohol in the wine and multiply it by 2. Multiply that total by the number of ounces you're drinking. Then multiply that answer by 0.8. For example, if you had an 8-ounce glass of a 10-percent alcoholic wine, the computations would look like this:

$$2 \times 10 \text{ (percent of alcohol)} = 20$$
$$20 \times 8 \text{ (ounces)} = 160$$
$$160 \times 0.8 = 128 \text{ calories}$$

47 The culprit for a lot of family strep throat problems may be stalking you on all fours right now. As many as 10 percent of pet cats and dogs are infection carriers, passing along the germ to children who snuggle with and kiss their furry friends. Even repeated doses of infection-killing drugs don't help—the kids go home from the doctor's office and get reinfected by a mere lick on the nose. Besides keeping an eye on pet smooching, your best bet is to have your pet checked by a vet; if it's a carrier, you needn't panic. Just make taking an antibiotic a family affair—Rover and Garfield included.

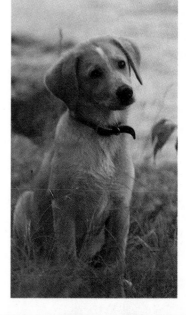

48 Ah, romance . . . the alluring candlelight, soft music, sparkling Spumanti and even more sparkling companion add up to a perfect atmosphere for—gluttony. Such environments can be so conducive to whetting the appetite that some people eat more than twice as much as usual, according to a study released by St. Luke's Hospital in New York City. This response is learned and therefore can be unlearned, according to the study. So if you're trying to slim down, avoid the distractions of elegant restaurants till you reach your goal.

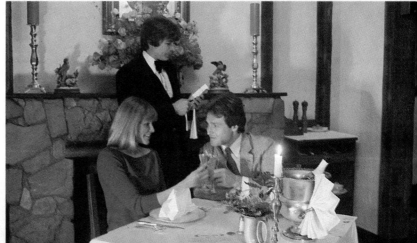

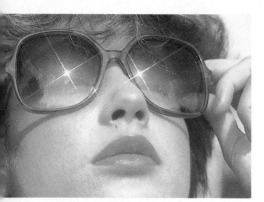

49

If it's summer and you're suddenly feeling kind of numb around the nose and mouth, don't panic—take off those large sunglasses. Many oversize sun-specs tend to be designed so that they press against a facial nerve, causing numbness. The cure is simple: Don't wear those shades; buy smaller ones.

50

If you're concerned about the amount of salt (sodium) in your food, here's some good news. You can eat many of the items you've been forsaking (and craving). The trick is to give them a 60-second bath first. The sodium content of water-packed, salt-added tuna can be reduced by as much as 79 percent if you run tap water over it for 1 minute and then let it drain. The same procedure flushes away 41 percent of the sodium in canned vegetables.

51

If too much talking on the telephone has reduced your free time to the hours you sleep, try making yourself less comfortable when you talk. If you usually slouch on the couch, plunk your bottom on a hard stool or the floor. Make eating, drinking or fingernail painting taboo until the phone's nestled safely back in its cradle. Face a clock, or stick your watch smack under your nose. Stick to the reason you or your caller called, and don't fly off on tangents. With one exception (the phone company), your relationships should improve.

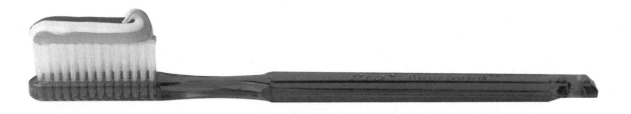

52

The calcium and phosphate in saliva replace minerals that decay destroys. But saliva can alter and turn against you, sometimes in surprising ways. Chewable vitamin C tablets are one culprit. A professor at Tufts School of Dental Medicine claims that chewable C's make saliva more acidic, eroding tooth enamel if left unneutralized. So, be careful: Brushing after supplementing is your best bet.

53

You probably shouldn't follow Granny's prescription for 100 or so good strokes with a hair brush every night. This might have worked for Granny—most women washed their hair less often back then, so they had a lot of oil to lubricate the brush bristles—but it could give your frequently washed and electrically dried hair the shaft. Splits and breaks are the only results of vigorous, repetitive brushing.

54

To protect your scalp from bristle scratches (they're not a major health problem, but they can hurt), buy only brushes with smooth, rounded bristle tips.

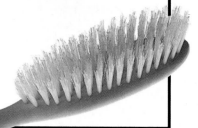

55

As many as 9,000 eye injuries a year result from playing racquet sports. (They don't call it squash for nothing!) Most injuries are preventable if you use a proper eyeguard. A lot of racquet sports establishments offer only the lensless, open-eye protector, however. Although these lensless eyeguards stop most injuries caused by the racquet itself, 95 percent of racquetball injuries are caused by the ball. Experiments have shown that an experienced racquetballer hits the ball at 127 miles an hour; at only 50 miles an hour racquetballs and squash balls distort enough to go right through the narrow eye opening of the so-called protectors, with disastrous results.

Ophthalmologists agree that the eyeguard that meets the highest safety specifications—the one you ought to use—is one with a polycarbonate lens (prescription or nonprescription), vented to decrease fogging, in a hingeless, wraparound frame.

56

Eat breakfast. Fourteen percent of Americans don't, but by waiting too long to break your overnight fast, you make your body think that it's starving. This slows your metabolism, which means that calories burn off more slowly. Translation: You don't get thin by skipping breakfast, and you could get fatter. Meanwhile, breakfast normalizes blood sugar levels during the morning, increasing your energy and alertness for the day ahead.

58

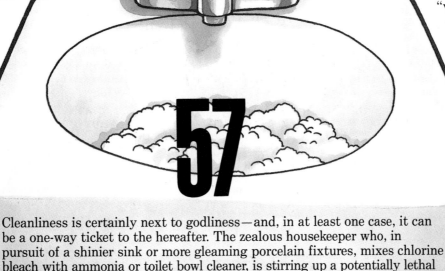

Chlorine can cause a ruckus when it comes to your underwear, too. Should you bleach those unmentionables of yours, beware of the potential for skin rash. The chlorine chemically alters elastic, and could give new meaning to the phrase "visible panty line" —the rash will be visible even when the panties are off.

57

Cleanliness is certainly next to godliness—and, in at least one case, it can be a one-way ticket to the hereafter. The zealous housekeeper who, in pursuit of a shinier sink or more gleaming porcelain fixtures, mixes chlorine bleach with ammonia or toilet bowl cleaner, is stirring up a potentially lethal result: deadly gas. Read the labels of commercial cleaning agents, and keep the antagonists apart.

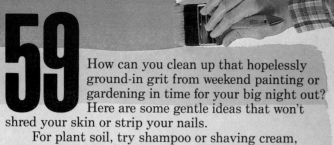

59 How can you clean up that hopelessly ground-in grit from weekend painting or gardening in time for your big night out? Here are some gentle ideas that won't shred your skin or strip your nails.

For plant soil, try shampoo or shaving cream, preferably unmedicated, and lather it away. To remove paint, try baby oil instead of turpentine. If the paint's oil based, it should slide right off. If you're going to be crawling around the innards of your car, lightly coat your hands with petroleum jelly to keep the grease off. Wear work gloves or use a rag when you need a nonslip grip, and use shampoo for cleanup. To remove ink splotches, put a drop of mild hydrogen peroxide on a cotton swab, then rub it on your skin. Rinse with water. If it's a really tough customer, try a little rubbing alcohol after using the peroxide.

60 Standing at a bar can be hard on the liver, but it's actually good for the back. If you must stand for a long time, wherever you are, it'll be much easier on your spine if you rest one foot higher than the other. Taverns all over the world have known this for centuries; that's what the brass foot rail is for. The same advice goes for airports or bus stations: Rest one foot on your suitcase to ease the strain on your back.

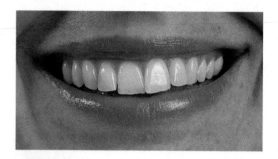

61 A growing number of dentists recommend brushing with baking soda and peroxide to fight periodontal (gum) disease. This could be a problem for some people with high blood pressure, however, as there are large amounts of sodium in baking soda. Answer: Keep the baking soda in the pantry and use Epsom salts instead. They'll do the same job without giving you a brush with danger.

62 If there weren't enough good reasons to stop smoking (we think there are *only* good reasons), here's another, aimed at the skyrocketing number of women puffers: Cigarette smoking brings an end to a woman's child-bearing years earlier than would occur naturally. A Danish study has shown that among women between the ages of 47 and 51, more heavy smokers (14 cigarettes a day) than nonsmokers had passed menopause, leading the scientists to believe that "cigarette smoking [is] a promoter of the menopause."

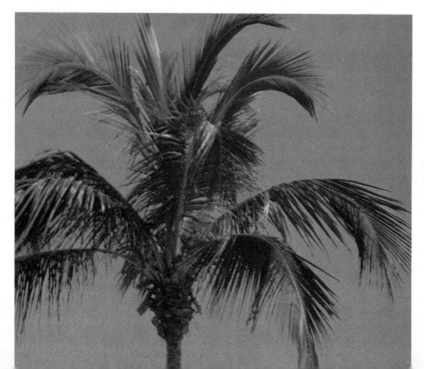

63 There are violent global outbreaks and skirmishes every day—inside the bodies of unsuspecting and vulnerable travelers. Before you leave the safety of home, call Worldwide Health Forecast (800-368-3531). This health hotline dispenses up-to-the-minute news on any nasty medical conditions around the world, along with health tips and guides to foreign medical facilities.

64

Sitting with one or both knees higher than your hips puts the least strain on your back. If you're driving, put the car seat forward enough to lift your knees up; if you're a passenger, cross your legs, or rest one foot on the transmission hump.

At the office, adjust your chair so your knees are raised, or put your feet up on a low stool. Just be sure your knees are bent so the soles of your feet rest flat on the stool. Don't extend your legs straight out; this position aggravates strain.

65

A piece of gauze, a jug of wine and . . . wow! There's something in wine that speeds up the healing process of certain skin ulcers, doctors say. By applying wine compresses for 15 minutes 4 times a day, people who had been trying to get rid of ulcerations for as long as 6 months saw them disappear in as little as 2 weeks.

66

Popping contact lenses into your mouth to wet them can spread to your eyes whatever germs are afloat in your saliva. Specifically, those people who are prone to cold sores from oral herpes are setting themselves up for a painful infection. Spend a few bucks for a wetting solution, instead of 10 to 50 times as much for doctor's visits.

67

Here's a new twist on an old exercise: Don't twist. The side-to-side upper body twisting that so many folks do in the belief that it will get rid of "love handles" and firm up the waistline is just so much wasted motion. Even more, it can cause injury to the tenacious twister. A slow twist loosens up the waist, side and stomach muscles, but doesn't do any firming or tightening. And a fast side-to-side can lead to pulled muscles or lower back pain. Better to apply resistance to the muscles you want toned—lifting weights is one sure way to do it.

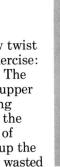

68

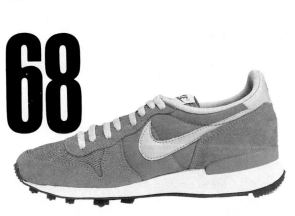

To avoid the unnecessary blisters that joggers' feet in new running shoes are heir to, wear the new pair around the house for a couple of weeks to introduce them casually to your tender tootsies. Then use them for another few weeks only for light training before taking your shoe on the road.

69

For 5 or 10 minutes, or whatever amount of time you can spare during the tensest part of your day, stop and take a humor meditation break, suggests Joel Goodman, Ed.D., director of the HUMOR project at the Sagamore Institute. Relaxing at your desk or any place where you can close the door on the outside world is fine. Then "meditate" —by reading a funny passage from a joke book or a novel or a humor notebook/scrapbook you keep for just such occasions. Or turn on a cassette of your favorite comedian, sit back and become one with the cosmic giggle. Experience the slightly Zen sound of one mouth laughing. Then return to work or chores or kids relaxed, refreshed and, somehow, renewed.

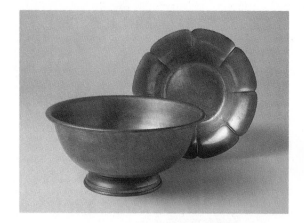

70 When you're about to partake of a repast served on pewter dinnerware, watch out: If the pewter was made before 1930, chances are good the lead content is high and that lead could be oozing its way into your food. You need only be wary of antiques and family heirlooms—modern pewter is lead free.

71 And while we're on the subject, don't leave leftover fruit juice or any kind of acidic food in the can once it's been opened. The lead solder that joins the can's seams can leach into the product.

72 Finally, our old noxious pal, lead, has one more leaching trick up its sleeve— this time it contaminates your household air. This potential toxin is released when the colored pages of newspapers and magazines are used to keep a roaring blaze going in your fireplace. The inks are loaded with lead just looking for a body to invade. The by-products of burning these coated sheets of paper can be especially harmful for children. Take the time to segregate the good stuff from the bad.

73 If you're being told you need an operation, but you're not sure and don't know where to turn, pick up the phone and call the Second Surgical Opinion Hotline. The number is 800-638-6833 (in Maryland, 800-492-6603). A trained volunteer will give you the names of surgeons in your locale, in the specialty you need, who have agreed to act as consultants.

74 Severe acne can make life a nightmare, but now there's a national hotline for acne sufferers. Call 800-235-ACNE (800-225-ACNE in California) for information on causes and cures.

75 Stomach difficulties can be scary propositions, especially if it's late at night or you're away from home. Enter Gutline, a telephone call-in service of the American Digestive Disease Society. By dialing 301-652-9293 on Tuesdays and Thursdays between 7:30 and 9:00 P.M. (EST), you and your tum will be connected to a gastroenterologist who will listen to your problems and discuss possible routes to recovery.

76 Raw meat juices can leak into the cracks of a wooden cutting board, setting up conditions for salmonella bacteria to breed; vegetables cut on the same board can pick up the bacteria. If you eat them raw, you could risk food poisoning. Use two cutting boards instead—one for meat, the other for veggies and fruit. (Use one side for chopping onions and garlic, the other side for less pungent foods.) Every so often, wash the boards with a solution of 1 tablespoon chlorine bleach per quart of water and wipe dry. You could also replace your wooden boards with plastic ones.

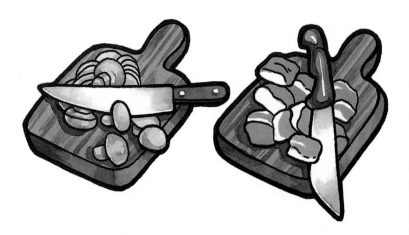

77

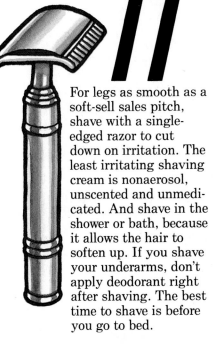

For legs as smooth as a soft-sell sales pitch, shave with a single-edged razor to cut down on irritation. The least irritating shaving cream is nonaerosol, unscented and unmedicated. And shave in the shower or bath, because it allows the hair to soften up. If you shave your underarms, don't apply deodorant right after shaving. The best time to shave is before you go to bed.

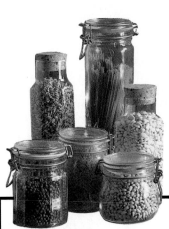

78

There may be a fairly painless way to stop smoking that's entirely nutritional. The way some researchers see it, the reason smokers want to keep smoking is because their urine carries nicotine out of their bodies. The more nicotine that goes out, the more the smoker wants to replace it.

Studies show that heavy smokers have very acidic urine; the higher the acidity, the more they smoke. And highly acidic urine ships that nicotine out of the body like an eager beaver. Smokers who wish to quit must make their urine less acidic and more alkaline, leading to greater nicotine retention and less smoking.

A simple shift in diet can help. Here's a list of alkaline (+) and acidic (−) foods to help you beat the butt.

Alkaline-Acid Effects of Some Common Foods			
Food	Amount	Alkaline (+) or Acid (−) Effect	Calories
Molasses	2 tsp.	+ 60.0	40
Lima beans, dried, shelled	⅛ cup	+ 42.0	91
Raisins	⅓ cup	+ 34.0	131
Figs, dried	1½	+ 33.0	83
Spinach	1 cup	+ 27.0	22
Brewer's yeast, dried	1 tbsp.	+ 17.1	35
Almonds	12	+ 12.0	88
Carrots	1 large	+ 11.0	40
Celery	2 stalks	+ 7.8	8
Grapefruit juice	½ cup	+ 7.0	43
Sweet potatoes	1	+ 6.7	175
Tomatoes	1 small	+ 5.6	20
Strawberries	12	+ 5.5	36
Mushrooms	7	+ 4.0	30
Apples	1 large	+ 3.7	90
Whole milk	1 cup	+ 2.3	145
Buttermilk	1 cup	+ 2.2	74
Onions	1	+ 1.5	23
Summer squash	1 cup	+ 1.0	17
Butter	2 pats	0.0	103
Honey	1 tbsp.	− 1.1	80
Whole wheat bread	2 slices	− 3.6	129
Peanuts	16	− 3.9	83
Cottage cheese	⅛ cup	− 4.5	28
Cheddar cheese	1 oz.	− 5.0	110
Brown rice	3 tbsp.	− 5.7	106
Buckwheat flour	2 tbsp.	− 7.1	77
English Walnuts	12	− 7.8	97
Codfish	¼ lb.	− 8.4	79
Lamb chops	2	− 9.7	260
Beef liver	¼ lb.	− 11.0	149
Beef loin	¼ lb.	− 11.0	385
Eggs	1	− 11.0	82
Chicken	¼ lb.	− 14.0	141
Lentils, dried	2 tbsp.	− 16.0	94
Wheat germ	2 tbsp.	− 20.0	76

79

Carbo-loading, the diet delight of runners, may also help people who suffer chronic pain. Researchers have found that combining the amino acid tryptophan with a diet high in complex carbohydrates (10 percent protein, 70 to 80 percent complex carbs) can reduce perception of pain. High-carbohydrate foods like whole grains and beans are believed to help transmit tryptophan to the brain. In concentrated doses, this substance has been used successfully to treat patients with severe pain who failed to find relief with more drastic painkillers.

Tryptophan tablets are available at health food stores, but no one really knows what the long-term effects are, so don't start downing them like popcorn. Besides, a high-carb diet naturally raises tryptophan levels in your body.

80

Have you spent 15 minutes a day in the bathroom with your best friends lately? Well, you should: If you don't take care of your teeth, they won't take care of you. Get two brushes, one for the morning and a fresh one for night. Small, soft brushes that won't scratch your gums and can dig into all the nooks and crannies are best. First, hold your brush at a 45-degree angle to the base of your teeth and massage the gum for a few seconds, then wiggle along the length of the tooth to the tip. It'll be tough at first, but try to get to the inside and outside of each tooth. And floss *after* brushing to avoid pushing debris back between the teeth.

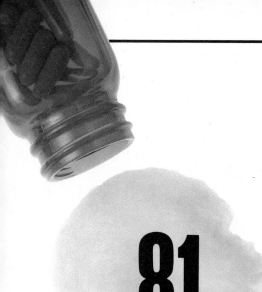

81

The cotton that's crammed into medication and vitamin bottles isn't doing you a bit of good. Get rid of it as soon as you open the container—otherwise, it will sit there and silently suck up enough of the ingredients or nutrients to diminish the pills' effectiveness. It will also trap germs from repeated handling and pass them on to your pills.

82

Ever wonder whether a cut heals better when it's kept covered and moist or exposed to the air to form a scab? One kind of bandage now on the market protects wounds better than gauze bandages and allows healing about 40 percent faster than air-exposed skin. Sold under the brand names DuoDerm, Tegaderm, OpSite and Vigilon, this nonstick dressing also seals the wound and keeps it moist.

83

Don't take antibiotics for the common cold—they kill bacterial infections but not the kinds of viruses that give you sneezes and sniffles. Plus, taking antibiotics when you don't really need them can make your body's bacteria resistant to the drugs, and trigger other possible side effects as well.

84

When you do need to take antibiotics, be sure you don't wash out the effects with the liquid you drink to wash them down. Milk can cancel out the medicinal benefits of certain antibiotics, and so can fruit juices. Stick with plain water instead.

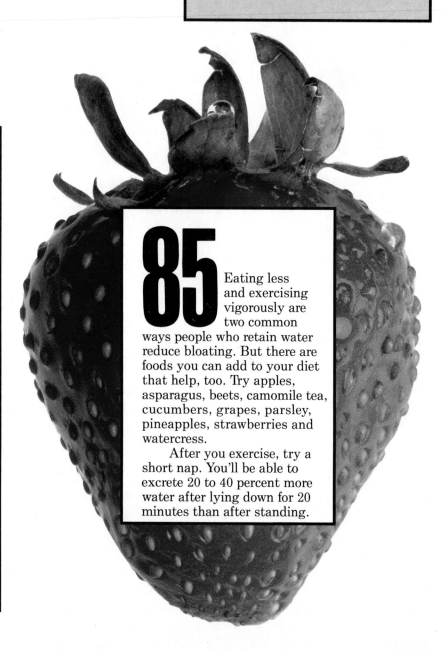

85

Eating less and exercising vigorously are two common ways people who retain water reduce bloating. But there are foods you can add to your diet that help, too. Try apples, asparagus, beets, camomile tea, cucumbers, grapes, parsley, pineapples, strawberries and watercress.

After you exercise, try a short nap. You'll be able to excrete 20 to 40 percent more water after lying down for 20 minutes than after standing.

86 Don't bother to gargle with aspirin to soothe a sore throat. Aspirin has to get into your bloodstream via your stomach to work, since it doesn't penetrate the skin or the throat lining. Stick to salt water instead.

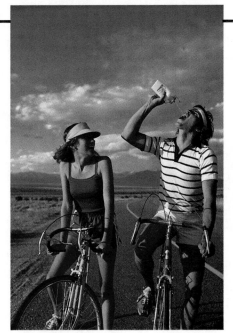

87 Taking a salt pill to counter the effects of heat and dehydration might be one of the worst things you can do. The old theory was that you lose lots of salt when you perspire, and it needs to be replaced. In truth, most of what your pores pour out is water, so the percentage of salt remaining in the body is higher, not lower. Taking a salt pill will only make matters worse. Water's the best remedy, with fruit juice a close second.

88 Taking pills is certainly no laughing matter, but it's very often a gag. Here's a simple trick to help: Swill your pill with about 3 ounces of water, tilting your head back as you swallow. If you're taking a lightweight capsule, tilt your head forward so the capsule floats to the back of your mouth. To add some gravity to the matter, take your pills standing up and remain standing for at least 90 seconds.

89 Now that salt's been put on the dietary nogoodnik list because of its ill effect on many people's blood pressure, America's ever-resourceful food processors and manufacturers have hopped on the antisodium bandwagon. Suddenly, phrases like "no salt" or "low sodium" are popping up on favorite foods stocked on supermarket shelves everywhere. But what do all those terms mean?
- "Sodium free" (also "salt free")—5 milligrams or less of sodium per serving.
- "Low sodium"—35 milligrams or less.
- "Moderately low sodium"—up to 140 milligrams.
- "Reduced sodium"—at least 75 percent of the sodium has been removed through special processing.

90 If you're an allergy or asthma sufferer whose symptoms flare up when you drive, you might need a mechanic more than a doctor. Seems an allergist in Louisiana couldn't figure out why one of his patients' wheezes and sneezes got worse on the road, so he sampled the air flowing from the air conditioner and discovered a thriving fungus. The prescription? A quick trip to the local garage for an air-conditioner cleanup was all it took to restore free breathing.

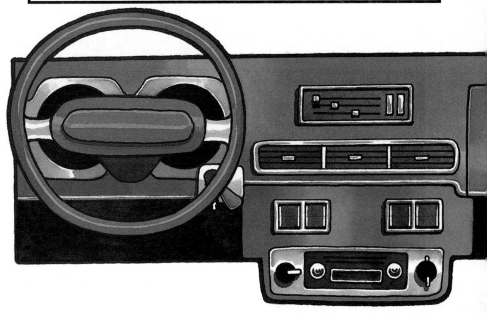

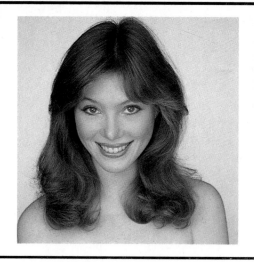

91 The best time to moisturize your face is at night. If you apply lotion before you leave the house, the water in your moisturizer will simply evaporate.

92 The National Health Information Clearinghouse, a service of the government's Office of Disease Prevention and Health Promotion, can put you in touch with people and organizations who can answer your specific health and medical questions—free of charge. Write the clearinghouse at P.O. Box 1133, Washington, D.C. 20013-1133.

93 Afraid to venture beyond telephone range of your family doctor? Fear no more. The American Academy of Family Physicians will send you its membership pages for the specific community you'll be traveling in (for example, not Southern California, but San Diego and Los Angeles) free on request. Contact them at 1740 West 92nd Street, Kansas City, MO 64114 (800-821-2512).

94 A New York City-based obesity specialist says there's a new metabolic miracle drug in the fight against fat! 100 percent natural and guaranteed to have no ill effects! Ladies and gentlemen— grapefruit juice! Luis Guerra, M.D., says that levels of cholecystokinin (CCK for short), a hormone produced and released in the small intestine when food enters it, causes the familiar feeling of fullness. Acidic liquids like grapefruit juice or unsweetened lemonade stimulate release of CCK. This process takes 20 minutes to work, so the doctor advises you to sneak in a glass of juice 20 minutes *before* sitting down to eat.

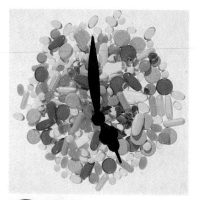

95 When it comes to vitamins and getting the optimum benefit, timing is everything.

The fat-soluble vitamins (A, D and E) and multivitamins ought to be taken along with the largest meal of the day, because that's when more fat is in the stomach to aid absorption.

The water-soluble vitamins (C and the B's) should be taken either during a meal or within a half hour before or after. Vitamin C is absorbed better if you take it in a few smaller doses during the day rather than one big dose.

96 The corrosive stomach acids that can cause heartburn could also be irritating your throat. If you suffer from mysterious hoarseness, scratchiness and a cough, try not to overeat; avoid fluids, especially alcohol, after meals; take an antacid between meals and at bedtime; and sleep with the head of the bed raised. Eighty-six patients who tried this program found that their throat problems disappeared; when they stopped it, most of them found that the problem returned.

97

Tofu—the soybean curd so popular today as a low-calorie, high-protein food—is sold loose in some stores, scooped right out of watery tubs like so many bars of floating soap. If the tub's refrigerated and the water's cold, buy away; if not, stay away. Food scientists have found that certain illness-causing bacteria set up camp on warm and wet protein foods— tofu among them. To avoid intestinal tofu-lishness, buy where you know it's cool, calm and collected, or purchase only the packaged kind.

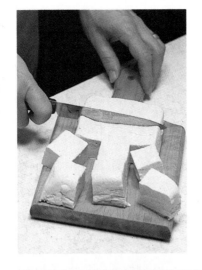

98

Using a salt shaker with a single small hole can make you use less salt, according to scientists at the University of New South Wales, Australia. Be careful, though—they also found that any hole smaller than 1/10 inch in diameter drove frustrated diners to drive their forks into the hole to try to enlarge it. Most salt shakers come ready-punched with holes, so try covering all but one with tape.

99

What's the best way to get rid of calluses? Bathe your feet in lukewarm water, mild soap and a skin-softening bath oil. Slough off the dead skin with a pumice stone rather than razorlike tools or acid-based foot softeners. Finish with a layer of moisturizing lotion like vitamin A cream. Buy shoes with a comfortable fit and keep your feet dry with powder or absorbent socks to reduce shoe friction and prevent more calluses from forming.

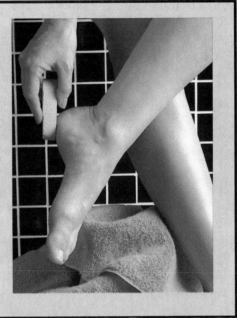

100

Plagued by in-grown hairs? You can prevent them by shaving more often but not as closely, using a sharp razor. Also, shave with the grain, not against it. Avoid pulling your skin taut when you shave.

Once you have ingrown hairs, try sloughing off the skin around them with a rough washcloth or a toothbrush before you shave. Release the hairs with a clean toothpick or sterile needle. Don't pluck them because they'll break through the wall of the hair follicle when they grow back, causing more irritation.

101

Sometimes putting events and situations into proper perspective is all that's required to eliminate stress. Whenever major league baseball pitcher Tug McGraw felt the bases-loaded, no-outs, bottom-of-the-ninth, tie-score jitters, he'd just consider the Snowball Theory, which goes something like this: "Millions of years from now the earth will drift farther and farther away from the sun and will become colder and colder, until it eventually resembles a giant frozen snowball. When that happens, will anybody care if Tug McGraw won or lost tonight's game?" Incidents seem a lot less life-or-death when you understand their cosmic significance—or insignificance.

9

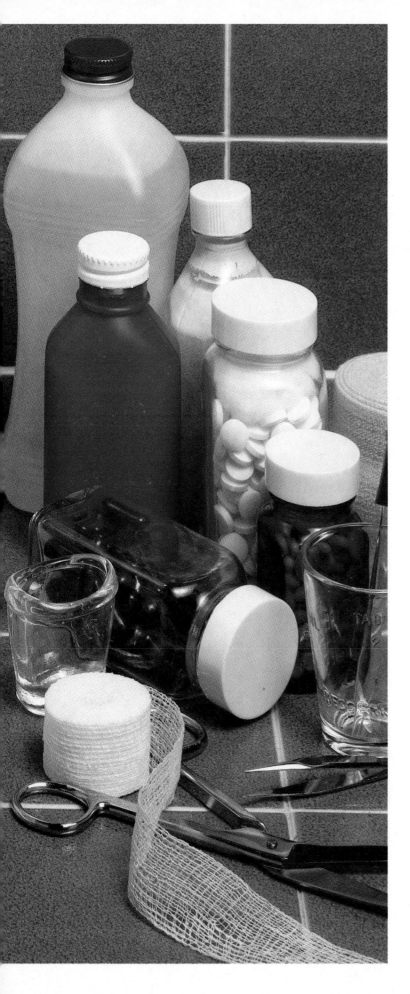

Emergency First Aid

Quick thinking, a cool head and a hopeful attitude can save a life—maybe yours.

E ven the most mundane items like old newspapers, broomsticks or common tap water can help save a life, but the greatest tool you have in administering first aid is a forceful, optimistic attitude. If you become shocked or panic-stricken at the sight of blood, your fear may communicate itself to the person you're trying to help and double his apprehension. If you can be calm, confident and decisive, there is a good chance the person will respond and start on a quick recovery. Besides, when was the last time you heard about a hysterical paramedic?

Sometimes first aid is the only help you need to give a person; at other times it is the preliminary step in emergency care, a stopgap measure used before professionals can get to the scene of an accident. In either case, remember that first aid is practical, not theoretical. There's no substitute for common sense, awareness and prevention in avoiding accidents, but knowing the right thing to do could save a life—maybe yours.

This chapter outlines the most common emergencies and the most effective techniques you can master, given a little practice. Of course, the more skilled you are, the better. Some skills—like rescuing a drowning person from deep water with life-saving techniques or using cardiopulmonary resuscitation on a heart attack victim—require special training, so they're not included here.

For easy reference, the highlights of first aid are given—how to recognize and treat each condition, and important how-to's. The yellow boxes represent "don'ts," or caution warnings— things you should never do in an emergency because they could result in severe injury.

There is one "do" we'd like to mention right here—look over the information in this chapter *now.* By familiarizing yourself with first aid techniques *before* an emergency, you can prevent panic—and maybe even a fatal mistake.

Bleeding

Most people have an instinctive revulsion to large amounts of blood. If you do, try not to let it paralyze you. Because the rapid loss of blood can be fatal, your first priority in *all* bleeding emergencies is to stop the flow quickly. If you suspect internal bleeding, get medical help. Even if a victim has suffered multiple fractures and has swollen and painful limbs, stop the bleeding first.

Venous bleeding is dark red and flows slowly and steadily; arterial bleeding is bright red and flows in quick spurts from the wound. Arterial bleeding is far more serious, but both can occur at the same time.

Stopping Nosebleeds

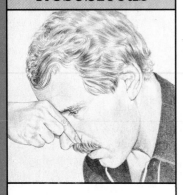

There are many ways to stop nosebleeds, but this is the best and safest.

Have the victim sit down and lean forward, with his mouth open to avoid choking on any blood that may get into the throat. Pinch the nose closed for 15 minutes, then release slowly. Repeat for 5 minutes if it's still bleeding. Then get a cold cloth or ice wrapped in a washcloth and hold it on the nose.

How to Apply Direct Pressure

1 Place any clean, absorbent cloth, such as sterile gauze or a towel, over the wound and press your hand against it. This will stop the bleeding but won't interfere with circulation. If no dressing is available, use your bare fingers. If blood soaks through the first cloth, add more cloths and continue to press steadily and firmly.

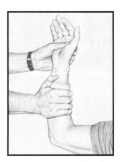

2 Elevate a bleeding limb above the level of the heart to reduce blood pressure. Continue to press firmly. If the bleeding stops or slows down, place a bandage over the dressing to hold it in place. Wrap the ends around the wound, pulling steadily to keep pressure on it. Then tie the knot directly over the wound.

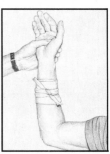

What Not to Do

Don't put any medication on a bad wound; it may cause an infection. Bleeding is nature's way of cleaning out the germs that may have entered through the wound, and any nonsterile ointment may foster more germs. And don't remove or disturb the dressing; you might tear off blood clots. Don't elevate a limb if you suspect a fracture because you might aggravate the injury with careless handling.

Recognizing and Treating Internal Bleeding

Symptoms and Signs	Action	What Not to Do
If pain seems greater than visible injuries, internal bleeding is a possibility. The symptoms are pain, tenderness, swelling and discoloration. The skin could be cold, pale and clammy; the pulse and breathing rapid; and the victim may be restless, dizzy, confused or unusually thirsty.	Keep the victim still. Give artificial respiration if necessary (see page 139), then get medical attention immediately. If the injury is minor, like a bruise or a black eye, simply put a cold compress on it.	Never administer fluids, no matter how raging the victim's thirst; if the stomach has ruptured, fluids will make the stomach contents leak into the abdominal cavity, which could cause infection. Don't move the person, if possible, because you can't always tell where injuries exist.

Arterial Pressure Points

If a wound on a limb is so severe that the bleeding can't be stopped by using direct pressure with elevation, add the pressure point technique. To stop the flow of blood to the wound, compress the main arteries against the bone at the points illustrated. Stop pressing when you've staunched the flow of blood.

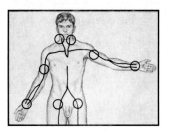

To control severe bleeding from the arm, press the brachial artery against the arm bone. The pressure point is located on the inside of the arm in the groove between bicep and tricep muscles, about halfway between armpit and elbow. Grasp this point with your thumb on the outside and the other fingers on the inside of the arm, then press firmly.

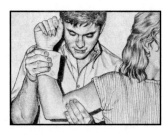

Pressing the femoral artery against the pelvic bone stops severe bleeding from the leg. If possible, put the victim flat on his back and put the heel of your hand on the thigh at the crease of the groin. It's harder to press this artery than the brachial artery, so keep your arm straight so you can comfortably apply your full body weight against the artery.

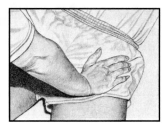

When to Use a Tourniquet

Tourniquets are a last-ditch attempt to stop bleeding that can't be controlled by direct pressure, elevation and arterial pressure. *They are to be used only in critical emergencies when there is a danger of bleeding to death.* Tourniquets completely cut off the circulation to a limb, so by applying one you risk losing the limb. Once applied, you can't remove it yourself and you *must* get medical attention.

A tourniquet should be at least 2 inches wide to effectively block circulation. You must wrap it tightly twice around the limb above the wound, then tie it in a half knot (like tying a shoelace). Place a stick or some other short, strong object on top of the half knot. Tie 2 more knots on top of the stick, then twist it tightly until the bleeding stops. Then treat the victim for shock (see page 153) or other injuries.

135

Bone and Muscle Injuries

Aside from having an X ray taken, there's no sure way to tell how severe an injury is; therefore treat any suspected sprain, strain or pull as a fracture.

How to Splint a Lower Arm Fracture

1 Gently put the victim's lower arm at a right angle across his chest with the palm facing toward the chest and the thumb pointing upward, as shown. Next, find a splint for the arm (almost anything rigid serves: boards, sticks, broom handles, corrugated cardboard, even newspapers or magazines wrapped around the arm). Pad the splint with a soft towel or cloth, then place the arm in it. The splint should extend well above and below the suspected fracture, running from the elbow to the wrist.

2 Once the splint is nestled against the arm, tie it in place above and below the break with anything available, from a belt to strips of an old sheet.

3 Support the splint with a sling. Slings can be made with a piece of any sturdy fabric about 3 feet square, folded diagonally in half. Put one end of it over the uninjured shoulder with the elbow nestled in the point of the triangle so that both ends are free. Elevate the hand about 4 inches above the level of the elbow and tie the ends of the sling together at the side of the neck, keeping the fingers free. Fold the point of the sling forward over the elbow and secure it to the outside of the sling, using a safety pin. If the victim complains of numbness, tingling or inability to move his fingers, loosen the ties; the splint is too tight.

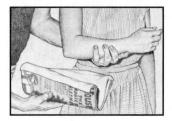

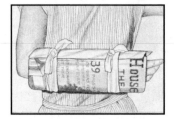

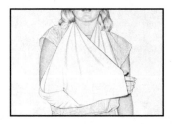

How to Bandage an Ankle

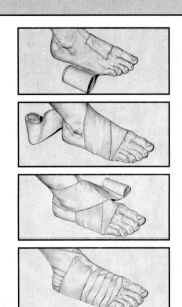

1 Lift the foot and anchor the bandage with 1 or 2 turns around the foot.

2 Bring the bandage diagonally across the top of the foot and around the ankle.

3 Diagonally wrap the bandage downward across the top of the foot and under the arch in a figure 8 pattern. Keep making figure 8's until the foot, ankle and lower leg are covered, keeping the toes free.

4 If you've done everything correctly and the bandage isn't so tight it cuts off circulation, secure the bandage with tape, clips or safety pins, or simply knot it.

Recognizing and Treating Bone and Muscle Injuries

Injury	Symptoms and Signs	Action	What Not to Do
Dislocation	When a bone becomes displaced from its joint—usually in the shoulder, hip, elbow, fingers or kneecap—it's dislocated. It looks misshapen, is extremely painful, swollen and discolored and quickly becomes immovable.	Splint and protect the affected joint, applying a sling if needed. Arm or leg joints should be elevated; hip or shoulder joints immobilized. Immediately following treatment, high-tail it to the nearest hospital.	Don't try to push the dislocated bone back in place. That's a tough job even for doctors, and unskilled handling can further damage the bone, nerves or blood vessels.
Fracture	Fractures are open (compound) or closed. (A fracture is open when the broken bone actually tears through the skin.) The injured person might have felt or heard a bone snap, or may feel the bone ends rubbing together. The injured area could be very painful, swollen, misshapen, or move abnormally.	If the victim isn't breathing, give artificial respiration (see page 139). Remove any clothing or shoes around the injured area (cut it away, if necessary), and keep that part of the body still. Stop any bleeding, then pad and splint the injured area, unless it's a broken back or neck or the person is unconscious. Treat for shock if necessary (see page 153). Then get help.	Don't wash the wound or apply any medication to it, and don't try to push back any part of a bone that protrudes through the skin. If at all possible, don't move the injured person, particularly if you suspect a neck or spine injury—the slightest movement could damage nerves and cause paralysis or death.
Sprain	Sprains happen when ligaments are stretched or torn, usually by overextending or twisting ankles, fingers, wrists or knees. The injured area could be painful, swollen, tender to the touch or discolored.	Keep the joint still. If the injury is to an ankle or knee, remove the shoe and apply ice wrapped in cloth for about 20 minutes to constrict the flow of blood and reduce the swelling. Repeat as needed. Elevate the leg to further reduce the swelling. If the wrist has been sprained, bandage and elevate it; if an elbow or shoulder, put it in a sling.	If a knee or ankle has been sprained, don't let the injured person walk. And don't apply heat to the affected joint for at least 24 hours after the injury; use ice. Don't assume any injury is a simple sprain. Be on the safe side and treat it as a fracture.
Strain	Strains occur when muscles are stretched beyond their normal range of movement, usually while performing strenuous activity. For instance, back strain is commonly caused by lifting heavy objects with the back bent but not the legs. The strained muscle may feel sore or knotted.	The victim should rest the affected muscle (a firm bed works wonders for strained backs). Apply ice or cold compresses immediately, then warm ones 24 hours later if needed. Aspirin or an aspirin-free painkiller like Tylenol should be used as little as possible—no more than 15 aspirin tablets per week or 8 Tylenols a day.	Don't move the affected muscle, and don't hesitate to call a doctor if the pain is severe.

Breathing Crises

Restoring breathing is always the first priority of *any* first aid: If a person isn't breathing, no other emergency aid will help. In most cases, we can survive only 6 minutes without oxygen. The most common cause of respiratory crisis is the tongue falling back and blocking the throat, so always check for that first.

How to Rescue a Drowning Person

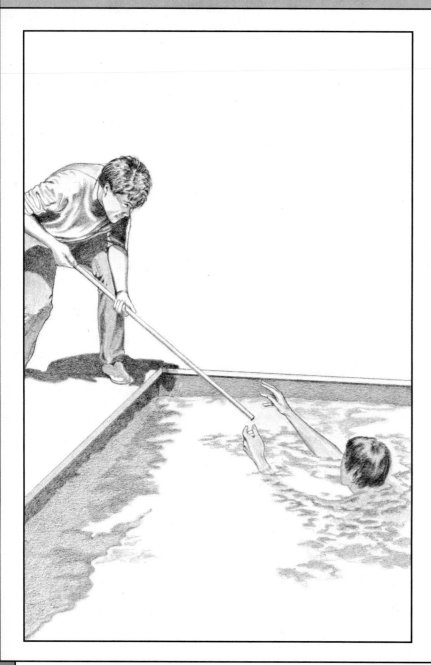

Drownings are the third-largest cause of accidental death. It is possible to save a drowning person even if you can't swim, but be careful not to overestimate your strength or ability. A drowning person may panic and drown both of you.

If the person is near the edge of the pool, dock or shore, extend anything that's handy, such as a life preserver, rope or a pole, and pull him in. If a boat is available and the victim is far away, row out to him and have him hang on to the back of the boat. If he can't hang on, *carefully* pull him into the boat; he could have internal injuries or fractures. If the victim is unconscious or you suspect a neck or back injury, put something wide and rigid like a surfboard under his back and haul him in. This prevents movement and possibly paralysis.

If the victim isn't breathing, begin artificial respiration (see opposite page) as soon as you can support the body on a hard surface. Don't waste time trying to empty the victim's lungs or stomach of water: People die from lack of air, not because they're bloated with water. Once the victim is breathing, turn him on his side and, if there's no spinal injury, extend the head backward to let water drain out. Keep the victim warm and get medical help quickly. Don't give anything to eat or drink.

How to
Give Artificial Respiration

1 Artificial respiration can be performed by almost anyone on any hard surface like a table, the deck of a boat or a sidewalk. If you're quite sure the person is unconscious, use your finger to quickly clear the mouth of anything blocking it. If the neck appears uninjured, put one hand under it and lift. Put the heel of your other hand on the forehead to tilt the person's head back as far as possible. If you think there's a neck injury, don't try this. Instead, put your forefingers and two middle fingers at the corners of the jaw by the earlobes and lift the jaw up.

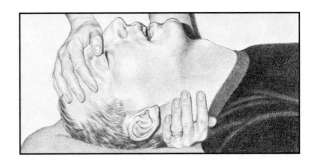

2 Pinch the nostrils together with your fingers or press your cheek against the victim's nose to keep the air you're going to force into his lungs from escaping through the nose. Now take a deep breath, clamp your mouth to the victim's to form a seal, then exhale. Repeat 3 more times, inhaling rapidly to allow as little air as possible to escape between breaths.

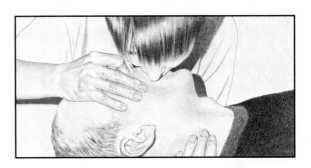

3 Take no more than 10 seconds to check for a neck pulse (see page 154). If there's a pulse but the person still isn't breathing, continue to blow into the victim's mouth once every 5 seconds until he starts breathing on his own. If there's no pulse, don't begin cardio-pulmonary resuscitation unless you're trained. Call an ambulance and paramedics immediately to continue treatment.

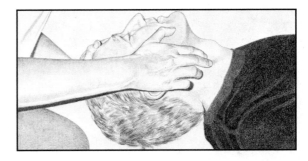

Helping Babies or
Small Children

Follow the same procedure to restore breathing in babies and small children, keeping in mind that they are smaller and more fragile. Don't tilt the head as far back as you would a larger child's or an adult's: Put one of your hands under the child's back and shoulders and lift slightly as shown here. That drops the head back and clears the throat. Then put your mouth over the child's mouth *and* nose, using small puffs of air to expand the chest every 3 seconds. Check for the pulse below the left nipple.

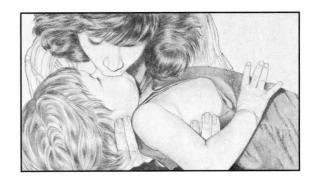

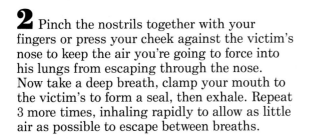

Burns

Burns from sun, hot substances or chemicals range in severity from first to third degree, depending on how many layers of skin are burned away. When only the outer layer of skin is damaged, as by mild sunburn or a brief scald, it's a first-degree burn. A severe sunburn or flash burns from gasoline are second degree if they damage several layers of skin and destroy nerve endings. A third-degree burn is even more painful: All layers of skin tissue have been destroyed by prolonged contact with heat or electricity.

You must be especially calm and comforting to a severely burned person: Aside from the searing pain, the victim could be hysterical about being scarred.

If you're not sure how severe the burn is, or whether the victim needs medical attention, use this simple rule: Any burn covering more than 15 percent of an adult's body or 10 percent of a child's requires immediate professional care. One hand, front and back, is about 1 percent of total body area, and an adult hand covers about 3 to 4 percent of a baby's body.

When Someone Catches on Fire

If someone's clothing has caught on fire, throw the person to the ground with the burning side uppermost. Smother the flames with a blanket, coat, tarpaulin or similar item, beating the flames *downward* —away from the head. If the face is burned, breathing problems may develop. After you've put out the flames, remove whatever you used to smother the flames and treat the victim for second- or third-degree burns.

Treating Chemical Burns

Affected Area	Action	What Not to Do
Skin	Inundate the burned area with gallons of running water for at least 5 minutes, using a garden hose, shower, sink or tub faucet or bucket. The longer a chemical's been in contact with the skin and clothing, the worse the burn, so flush it out quickly and get the clothing off. If the chemical container's available, check it for any first aid directions. Cover the burn with a clean cloth, then get medical attention.	Never apply antiseptics, ointments or sprays; they can complicate or increase the severity of the burn.
Eyes	Flush out the eye very quickly; damage can occur within 1 minute. Wash the eye from the inner corner outward: This avoids getting the chemical that's in one eye into the other. Cover the eye, lid closed, with a clean dressing, and get medical assistance, preferably from an eye doctor.	Eyes are one of our most fragile organs, so the warnings about the use of ointments and cotton apply triply: Cotton fibers will stick to the wound and eyelashes, and ointments may further inflame the eye. Don't let a burn victim rub the eyes; that could increase the damage.

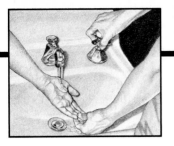

Immediate Aid for
First- and Second-Degree Burns

As quickly as possible, put the burned area under cold water from the sink or apply a cold (not icy) wet cloth until the pain subsides. Gently blot the burn dry, then apply dry, sterile gauze or a clean cloth as a bandage. Don't apply butter, grease, ointment, lotion or spray. They could increase the possibility of infection. Don't break the blisters. If the burn is large or severe, get help.

Recognizing and Treating Burns

Type	Symptoms and Signs	Action	What Not to Do
First Degree	The burned area is red, swollen and painful, but the skin isn't broken. There aren't any blisters, and healing is rapid.	Immediately put the burned part under cold water or apply a cold compress, such as a clean towel or handkerchief soaked in cold water, then cover the burn with clean bandages to protect it against further irritation or rubbing.	Don't put butter or grease on the wound, despite popular wisdom—they could cause infection.
Second Degree	The burn looks red, blotchy or deeper than a first-degree burn, since more than one layer is damaged. Blisters form, and swelling may persist for several days. The skin might appear wet and oozy due to plasma leaking through the damaged layers of skin.	Proceed exactly as for a first-degree burn. If the arms or legs have been burned, keep them elevated to reduce swelling, then get medical help. If the person has been burned around the face, breathing problems may develop, so be prepared to administer artificial respiration (see page 139).	Don't use ice or icy water. Don't break the blisters or apply any ointments, antiseptic sprays or home remedies. Don't use cotton balls when bandaging the wound; they will only deposit irritating fibers that may cause infection.
Third Degree	The burned area looks charred and white. All skin is destroyed. There is little or no pain if nerve endings have been destroyed.	Check the victim's breathing and be prepared to give artificial respiration. 　Put a cold cloth or cool water on the burn to relieve pain, if any, then cover the burn with a thick, sterile bandage. Then call an ambulance immediately. Elevate burned body parts, if possible. If the victim is unconscious and the burns permit it, turn the victim on one side to allow fluids (blood, vomit, saliva) to drain from the mouth to prevent choking. Treat for shock if necessary (see page 153). Above all, keep calm and reassure the victim: Third-degree burns are highly traumatic.	Don't use ice water, ointments or sprays. Don't remove any clothing stuck to the burn—that's for a doctor to do. Don't try to give an unconscious person water: Swallowing is not an automatic function like breathing or the heartbeat, and he could choke.

Choking

Choking is the ninth-largest cause of accidental death. According to Henry J. Heimlich, M.D., the Cincinnati doctor who in 1974 invented the maneuver that bears his name, 90 percent of choking victims are eating when the problem occurs, and 98 percent of people who fall unconscious and die in or near restaurants have choked to death.

The basis of the Heimlich maneuver is simple: Despite a choking victim's gasps, a lot of air remains in the lungs. The maneuver forcibly elevates the diaphragm, compressing the lungs and expelling this air, and the obstruction, at great pressure. About a quart of air explodes out of the mouth in a quarter of a second if the technique is performed correctly, says Dr. Heimlich. If a person is unconscious and you can't inflate his lungs with artificial respiration because of the obstruction in his throat, apply the maneuver.

How to Apply the Heimlich Maneuver

Stand behind the victim and wrap your arms around his waist, allowing the victim's head, arms and upper torso to hang forward. Make a fist and place the thumb side against his upper abdomen, slightly above the navel and below the rib cage, as shown. Now grasp your fist with the other hand and press inward with a quick upward thrust. Your fist is actually thrusting upward into the diaphragm, compressing the air still in the lungs and forcing it through the windpipe. Repeat several times if necessary.

If the victim is sitting, stand or kneel behind him and perform the maneuver exactly as if he were standing. If the victim is lying on the ground, don't waste valuable time trying to raise him; instead, roll him on his back and straddle him. Place the heel of one hand on top of the other, as illustrated, and press quickly upward. Don't try to kneel next to the victim, because you can't thrust directly upward in that position, and you could rupture the liver or the spleen.

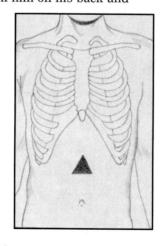

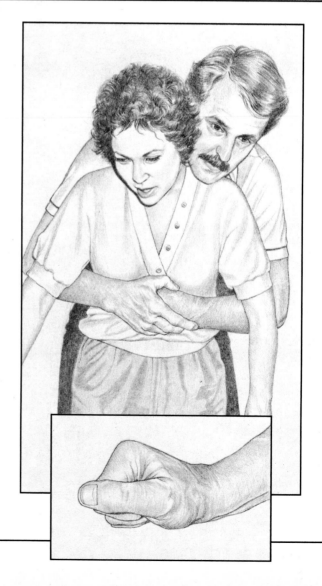

Signs of Choking

A choking victim gasps and coughs, has noisy, labored breathing and is unable to speak. He will turn very pale, even bluish, as oxygen is cut off to body tissues. The victim may collapse or become unconscious. (Dr. Heimlich has devised a commonsense sign to indicate when you're choking, since a choking victim can't speak: Grasp your throat with your hand.)

Helping Yourself

The maneuver is exactly the same if you must perform it on yourself: Put the thumb side of your fist into your upper abdomen, grasp it with the other hand and press upward quickly. Or you can lean your upper abdomen against the back or edge of a chair, sink, table or porch rail and press against it in the same place.

Helping Pregnant or Obese Victims

Place your fist on the middle of the breastbone, not on the upper abdomen. Give 4 quick thrusts, but be careful not to squeeze with your arms; otherwise, you could endanger the pregnancy. Be sure to press with enough force if the person is obese.

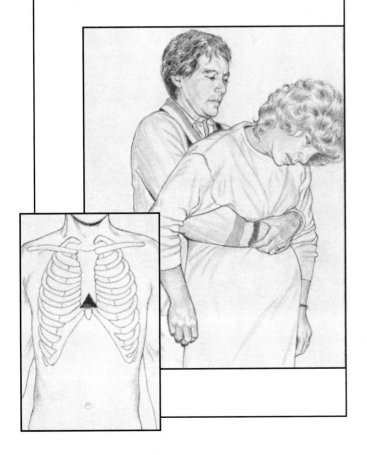

Helping Babies or Small Children

Be gentle: Babies are far more fragile than adults. There are 2 ways to save an infant or small child, and neither way uses as much force as you'd use on an adult. The first is to hold the child seated in your lap. Reach around and place the index and middle finger of both hands against the baby's upper abdomen (above the navel and below the ribcage) as shown.
Press inward with a rapid thrust. Or you can place the infant face-up on a firm surface and perform the maneuver, again using just the index and middle finger of both hands.

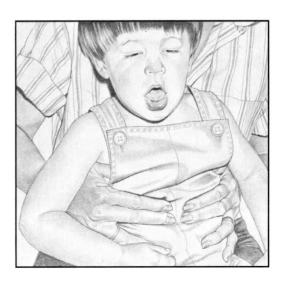

Electric Shock

Electricity can knock you down, render you unconscious and stop your breathing or heartbeat if it enters your body. The electric current heats up the body as it courses through, looking for an exit. The current usually travels via the bones and nerves, but it can fan out into the underlying tissues and cause widespread damage, even though all that's visible are small marks where the current entered and exited.

Don't directly touch a person who's still in contact with electric current—you could get a shock, too. Wait until the electricity has been turned off or you can remove the source. (Someone who has been struck by lightning can be touched immediately.) But act quickly! The less time a victim stays in contact with the current, the better his chances of survival.

Immediate Aid for Electric Shock

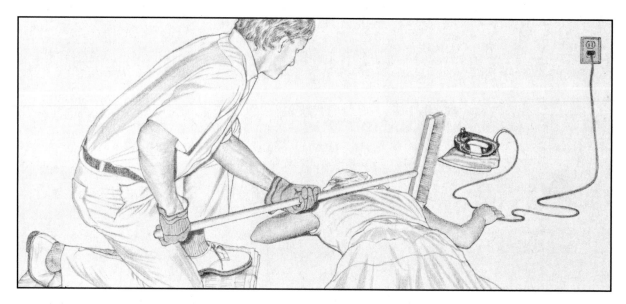

1 Try to turn off the electric current by removing the fuse, pulling the main electrical switch or calling the power company and asking them to cut it off. If you can't turn off the source, get the person away from the current. Make sure you are standing on something *dry* like a piece of wood, a newspaper, a blanket or, better yet, a rubber mat. Wear dry, insulated gloves, if you have them.

2 Get something long, sturdy and nonconducting, like a wooden broom handle or a plastic mop. Carefully push the person away from the current. If you can't move the victim, pull or push away the electrical source.

3 Immediately check the person's breathing and begin artificial respiration if necessary (see page 139). Get medical attention immediately, and remember even the tiniest burn marks may mean severe injuries.

Select a Safe Tool to Save the Victim

You come down from the shower in the morning and find your spouse face down on the floor, clutching a smoking toaster. Your first impulse is to rush over to help, but that impulse could electrocute you! *Don't* rush over and touch the person or the appliance: The human body is 75 percent water, and a fairly good electrical conductor.

Instead, either quickly shut off the electricity or find an electrical nonconductor in your kitchen, like a broom handle, plastic mop handle or wooden chair. Use it to push the toaster away (see opposite page). *Never* use anything wet, even a nonconductor. If in doubt about any object, don't use it! Find something else you're sure about.

Electrical Conductors

Anything metal is an excellent conductor of electricity, even anything *containing* metal, like an umbrella or a rake with a metal head and a wooden handle. Vacuum cleaners, lamps, guns, shovels, and car, bicycle or machine parts are also good conductors, and could transfer the shock to you.

Electrical Nonconductors

Wooden or plastic broom handles, mop handles and rakes don't conduct electricity too well. In fact, any long wooden object is safe—such as shelves, boards, sturdy sticks, fence posts, oars or canes. Rubber objects will work as well, as long as the object is long and stiff enough to prevent accidental contact.

Preventing Shocks

Keeping kilowatts from becoming *killer*-watts is primarily a matter of handling electricity with care. Begin by making sure all outlets, switches and appliances are located where they cannot be touched from the bath, shower or sink. Also be sure that appliances are permanently grounded—as in the installation of electric ranges and clothes dryers—or that they have a three-prong grounding plug. In addition, be sure to cover all unused wall sockets with protective tape, plates or blank plugs.

If your home is new, you might have built-in protection. The National Electrical Code now specifies that all new homes have a "ground-fault circuit interruptor." This device is installed in your home's circuit box or in designated outlets. It automatically cuts the power off when it senses the electricity isn't flowing where it should. If your home is not new, consider installing one. The device is available in most hardware stores.

These protective steps will cut the odds of electric shock, but here's how to handle some situations that might occur.

- What if you smell burning plastic or notice flickering lights?

   Immediately call a technician to check your household wiring. Often this problem is caused by overloading a particular, conveniently located circuit. In this case, simply redistribute your appliances.

- What if toast in the toaster starts to fume like a volcano?

   Never, ever, stick anything metal like a fork or knife into the appliance's guts while it's plugged in! Unplug it, or use wooden tongs to fish the crisped toast out.

- What if your hair dryer or other appliance falls into a tub or sink full of water?

   Don't touch the appliance or put your hand in the water; the water is now carrying an electrical charge. If your hands are wet, dry them, then unplug the appliance and don't use it again until it's been checked out by an electrician. It's probably been short-circuited, and you might have to throw it out.

- What if you want to make an electrical repair or replace a lighting fixture?

   First, turn off the current at the breaker or fuse box. Carefully complete the repair job. When you've finished, you will have to turn on the electricity again to see if you've succeeded at your work. At this time, be sure you are not using a metal ladder. Further protect yourself by standing on layers of newspaper or on a rubber mat for insulation.

- What if you receive a shock when you touch an electric appliance?

   Cease using it immediately. Make sure the appliance is properly grounded by checking that the screw fastening the green grounding wire has not become loose. If the screw is tight and shocking persists, other grounding locations in the appliance must be checked by a qualified electrician.

Foreign Objects

Splinters are a perennial affliction, but in most cases, they will come out easily. If the splinter looks too big, or the wound is serious or infected, don't attempt any first aid—just get medical attention.

This applies doubly to the eye. Eyelashes, cinders or small bugs can be blown or rubbed into the eye. These small particles may be extremely irritating to the eyeball and could scratch it or become embedded. If you see that the particle is really embedded, cover both eyes with clean, sterile bandages and get the person immediate medical help. Don't try to remove the particle.

How to Remove a Particle from the Eye

1 Wash your hands thoroughly with soap and water, and examine the eye in good light. Pull the upper eyelid down over the lower lid, then let it slide back. This will produce tears and might flush out the particle. If there is an eyedropper handy, fill it with warm water and squeeze over the eyeball to flush out the particle.

3 If you can't find the irritant, it might be underneath the upper lid. Get the person to look down while you place a cotton swab or wooden matchstick across the upper lid and gently fold the lid up over it.

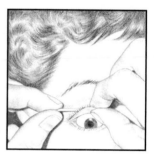

2 If the particle resists flushing, have the person look up while you pull the lower lid down. If you can see the object, pick it off with the corner of a moistened, clean cloth, handkerchief or paper tissue.

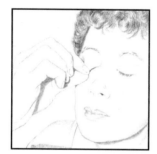

4 If you can see the particle, pick it off with the clean, moistened cloth, handkerchief or paper tissue. If you can't see it, cover both eyes with soft pads to prevent eye movement, and get medical attention.

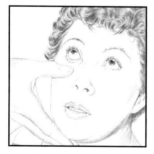

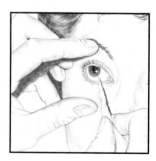

What Not to Do

Don't let the person rub his eye—he could scratch it, and the eyeball could become infected. Don't use cotton swabs to pick particles off the eyeball; their loose fibers will come off and stick. And never try to remove *anything* embedded in the pupil (the dark spot in the center of the iris) or in the white of the eye—these are very sensitive portions of the eye, and scratching them could result in permanent damage.

How to Remove Splinters

If you are near a source of warm water, soak the skin surrounding the splinter for 5 minutes. This will improve the circulation to the area and, more important, help mobilize the entire immunological system against any infection. Then sterilize tweezers by passing them through a flame or by dipping them in boiling water or rubbing alcohol. Now gently pull the splinter out.

If the splinter is embedded just beneath the skin, lift it out with the tip of a sterilized needle, then wash the injured area with soap and water. If the splinter is too deep to reach easily, let a doctor remove it.

How to Remove a Fish Hook

Catching a fish hook in the skin is quite common. Often, just the point of the fish hook enters, and it can easily be removed by backing it out. But if the hook goes deeper and the barb becomes embedded in the skin, it's best to have a doctor remove it. Bandage the hook so it can't dig in further, then get medical attention.

If medical help isn't readily available and you have the proper tools, you can remove a fish hook yourself. If the hook goes deep enough so that the barb is stuck in the skin, just push the hook through the skin until the barb emerges. Cut off the barb with pliers or clippers, then carefully back out the rest of the hook. Clean the wound with soap and water, cover it with a bandage, then see a doctor. Fish hooks aren't especially hygienic, so there's a real possibility of infection or tetanus.

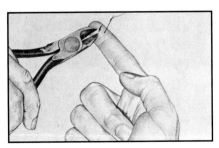
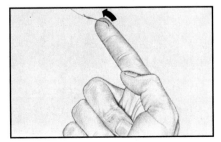

Heart Attacks

Heart attack is one of the few genuinely life-threatening emergencies that may occur with few or no warning symptoms, and no direct first aid possible (unless you know how to administer cardiopulmonary resuscitation). Still, recognizing a heart attack when it occurs, keeping the victim calm and comfortable and calling an ambulance may save a life.

A heart attack occurs when the blood supply to the heart is cut off for some reason—for instance, a clot in a blood vessel. Deprivation of oxygen-rich blood may cause irreversible brain damage in 6 minutes or less.

Heart attacks can be difficult to diagnose. The victim may or may not have a history of heart trouble, and an attack could occur without warning. The victim may or may not lose consciousness, and the degree of pain the person experiences is no reliable guide to the seriousness of the attack. Some heart attacks are even mistaken for indigestion!

Helping Yourself

If you feel you're having a heart attack and there's no one to help you, get on the phone and call an ambulance and paramedics immediately. Tell them the problem, and that you need oxygen. Then get comfortable, preferably propping yourself up with pillows. Loosen any tight clothing, especially around the neck, keep warm and don't eat or drink anything.

Recognizing and Treating Heart Attacks

Symptoms and Signs	Action	What Not to Do
The person may feel persistent central chest pains, usually under the breastbone, as though his chest is caught in a vise. The pain usually spreads to the shoulders and arms, especially the left arm, or to the neck, jaw, midback or abdomen. The victim may be weak, gasping, short of breath; the skin could be pale or the lips and fingernails blue. He could be sweating profusely and be nauseated or vomiting.	Check to see whether the person is wearing an emergency medical identification bracelet or necklace, or is carrying a card in his wallet saying he's had heart trouble. If the victim is unconscious, use artificial respiration (see page 139), *then call an ambulance and request oxygen.* If the person is conscious, gently put him in what he feels to be a comfortable position, usually sitting up or propped up on pillows so he can breathe more easily. Loosen tight clothing, particularly around the neck (remove neckties or bow ties immediately). Keep the victim warm, then call an ambulance or, if you must, take him to the hospital, transporting him gently.	Never initiate cardiopulmonary resuscitation to restart the heart unless you're certified to do so. CPR requires that you repeatedly pump the victim's breastbone vigorously; if you don't know what you're doing, you can cause severe internal damage. Don't give the victim anything to eat or drink.

CPR: The Miracle You Can Learn

Daring television paramedics have firmly established in everyone's mind the idea that cardiopulmonary resuscitation (CPR) is a miraculous means of snatching life from the jaws of death. It *is* a miracle: The second stage of cardiopulmonary resuscitation actually revives the heartbeat of someone whose heart has stopped—someone clinically dead—using mouth-to-mouth breathing and vigorous rhythmic chest compression. But only those people who have taken courses in CPR based on standards set by the American Heart Association or the American Red Cross should attempt this life-saving technique.

The most recent polls suggest that approximately 24 million people have been qualified to perform CPR. If you wish to learn CPR, you can take a simple 3- to 4-hour course or a far more detailed 9-hour course that includes training in how to remove obstructions from the heart attack victim's mouth and throat, resuscitation teamwork and techniques to use on infants and children as well as adults. Call the local office of the American Heart Association or the American Red Cross for details on classes. Any of these courses entitles you to a card certifying you to perform CPR, good for 1 or 2 years.

Poisoning

The chemical products that make our lives easier can hurt children: Up to 70 percent of all poisonings happen to children under 5. Vigilance and prevention—watching children closely (especially before meals, when they're hungry) and keeping all toxic substances high out of reach *and* locked up—are the best antidotes.

Conduct a poison tour of your home with your children, pointing out how even the most common products, like dishwashing detergent, can hurt them. If your child responds to a symbol like the bright green "Mr. Yuk," get some stickers from a poison control center and teach your child he means "NO!"

In case of poisoning, call your regional poison control center, rather than your neighborhood poison center. Regional centers have more up-to-date information and keep an experienced staff on duty 24 hours a day, 365 days a year.

Finally, try to remain calm. Often poisonings are not as serious as they look: One busy regional center reports that the only treatment 80 percent of its patients need is a strong shot of reassurance.

Meet Mr. Yuk

The ugly green face above probably caught your eye as soon as you turned to this page. Your 3-year-old will notice it, too, but will it prevent a poisoning? Don't count on it. There's simply no substitute for parental responsibility, supervision and teaching. No symbol can prevent poisonings; although Mr. Yuk is probably the most effective poison symbol ever created, he can only create an *awareness* of the poisons. Mr. Yuk is only a tool in an educational process that depends on how well you can inform your child.

Immediate Aid for Poisoning

Symptoms of poisoning vary tremendously, but there are definite clues to follow: Ask the victim or any observers what was swallowed, and check for any containers lying around. Victims of poisoning might suddenly vomit or have unusual pains, burns around the mouth or unfamiliar odors on their breath.

The first—and often only—action to take is to call the regional poison control center, prepared to offer the following information: the victim's age; what was ingested and how much (if you know); when it was taken; whether the person has vomited; estimated time required to reach the nearest medical facility. If you don't know where the nearest treatment center is, the poison control center will locate it for you, send an ambulance to your home and alert specialists at the treatment center or hospital. If the victim should vomit spontaneously before help arrives, make sure he doesn't choke. Scoop any vomited material into a plastic container and take it for laboratory analysis, along with the poison container.

What Not to Do

Don't induce vomiting unless the poison center suggests it—and then use syrup of Ipecac (available in drugstores).

Don't give the victim any fluids, especially if he's unconscious: Acidic juices may combine with the poison to trigger a chemical reaction and, contrary to popular opinion, diluting may actually inflict harm by spreading the toxin.

Ignore advice in pamphlets, brochures and even the best first aid manuals: Poison control is a new and rapidly changing field; often last year's wisdom is this year's folly. Don't follow the antidotes listed on containers, either: They could be outdated and dangerous.

Misleading Labels

Don't believe everything you read—labeling on many products is incomplete, erroneous or missing altogether. Federal law states that only extremely toxic products need warning labels that list the toxic ingredients. Even when a list of ingredients is provided, it could be obsolete, so antidotes on labels could also be useless or even hazardous. A recent study of product labels by the New York City Poison Control Center found 80 percent were inaccurate for these reasons. Even the most up-to-date labels recommend diluting the poison with water or other liquids on the assumption that this would weaken the toxic solution's effects. Poison centers explain that dilution could be dangerous because it can spread the poison.

Industrial-strength cleaners may have directions that are hopelessly complex or outdated, like this antidote from the label of a toilet bowl cleaner:

"Drink a teaspoonful or more of magnesia, chalk or small pieces of soap, softened with water in milk or raw egg white."

Why Regional Centers Are Best

Warning: Neighborhood poison control centers may be hazardous to your health. A recent survey found that 60 percent of the more than 400 poison control centers in the U.S. gave out inadequate or even dangerous advice. The regional centers that are members of the American Association of Poison Control Centers (AAPCC) have the best information available and are staffed by full-time paid professionals, not volunteers. Since the person who answers any center's phone determines how a case is treated before a doctor is called, you should call the most reliable, experienced source of information.

The AAPCC uses a computer-generated database, called Poisindex, of more than 400,000 products, their ingredients and the best antidotes. The information is updated 4 times a year. Poisindex has an informal contract with the major manufacturers of chemical products to list any new products or changes that might not be on the label—and 6,000 new products are authorized for sale each year by the U.S. Food and Drug Administration.

You need not automatically dismiss your local poison center, however. It could subscribe to the constantly changing association standards. Before any emergency occurs, check out local poison control centers. Here's what to look for: Is it staffed by a nurse, pharmacist or physician on each shift on a regular, full-time basis? Is the center open around the clock every day? Does it keep a written record of a victim's name, age, address and phone number for use as a medical and legal record? Only if the center meets your standards should you enter its number on your emergency phone list.

Preventive Tips

- Look up the number of the *regional* poison control center nearest you and keep it handy. Don't call just any center you find listed in the phone book; it will not necessarily be reliable.

- Keep a bottle of syrup of Ipecac (to induce vomiting) on hand for each family member.

- Aspirin is the main culprit in child poisonings, so keep it and all other medications out of reach, *always* in child-proof containers and preferably locked in a cupboard.

- Don't take any medication in the presence of children: They love to imitate adults. When you give a child medicine, don't call it candy.

- Make sure all medicines and household products are clearly labeled and in their original containers.

- Keep foods and household substances separate, and dispose of any outdated or unwanted product by washing it down the sink or toilet. Thoroughly rinse out the container, then throw it away.

Seizures

Seizures are brought on by disturbances in the brain's electrical activity. They look quite frightening, but they usually don't cause any serious problems by themselves. Injuries may result if the person falls or slams into surrounding objects while the seizure is in progress.

What Causes Seizures

Contrary to popular belief, seizures aren't limited to epileptics and people attacked by rabid, foaming beasts. All of us have a seizure threshold, based on the balance of the brain's electrical system. When one part of the brain fails to act in unison with the rest, a seizure could result.

Any number of stimuli could push the brain's neurons over that threshold, but high fever due to acute infections, physical injuries or organic illnesses of the brain and spinal cord top the list. Poisoning, drug withdrawal, hyperventilation, dehydration and vitamin and mineral deficiencies can also cause seizures. Seizures are so common in infants that they have been called "fifth-day fits."

All seizures are temporary. Keep in mind that the seizure is just a symptom, and is usually more frightening than dangerous.

Recognizing and Treating Seizures

Symptoms and Signs	Action
Seizures may begin with muscle rigidity, followed by jerking and twitching. When the muscles are rigid, the person may stop breathing, lose control of his bladder and bowels or bite his tongue. His face and lips could look bluish from lack of oxygen. Saliva may foam or drool from the mouth, the person may cry out and his eyes may roll upward.	Your main objective is simply to prevent the person from injuring himself. Try to catch him if he falls, especially protecting the head. Clear a space around the person, moving away hard objects like tables and chairs. Try to slip a pillow, blanket or something soft under his head so it isn't injured during the seizure. Loosen tight clothing if you can, and watch his breathing. You might have to restore breathing by artificial respiration (see page 139). When the seizure subsides, be comforting. The person is likely to feel very embarrassed, drowsy and confused. Look carefully for any injuries and tend to them. Keep the victim lying on one side (or turn his head) to allow fluids to drain from the mouth. Stay with the person until he's recovered, and get medical help, especially if another seizure occurs or if the victim is a pregnant woman.

What Not to Do

Don't try to hold the person still; his muscles could tear.

Don't throw cold water on his face or put anything in his mouth, despite what you may have heard.

Someone having a seizure experiences very little physical feeling, so throwing cold water in his face will have no effect at all. In fact, if the water gets into his lungs, he could choke to death! The jaws of someone undergoing a seizure can be incredibly powerful; they can break sticks and even fingers. Once an object has been broken off in the mouth, there's additional danger that the victim will choke on it.

Shock

Shock occurs when the amount of blood and oxygen being pumped to tissues plummets due to serious injury such as heart problems, infections, burns, fractures or breathing problems. So in addition to treating someone for a heart attack, fracture or whatever, you must treat for shock. Shock may be even more life-threatening than traumatic injury.

A Solution for Shock

In 1 quart of cool water, mix 1 level teaspoon of salt and ½ level teaspoon of baking soda. Give an adult or a child over 12 years old ½ cup (4 ounces), a young child ¼ cup (2 ounces) and a baby under 1 year old ⅛ cup (1 ounce) *slowly* over a 15-minute period.

Recognizing and Treating Shock

Symptoms and Signs	Action	What Not to Do
The skin of someone in shock can look pale, even blue (because of oxygen deprivation), and be moist and clammy. The person could feel very weak and be extremely thirsty, restless or anxious. His pulse could be too fast and weak, and he could be vomiting. Eventually, the shock victim's eyes will have a dull, sunken look, with dilated pupils, and his skin will look blotchy or streaked.	Check the victim for any breathing difficulties (see page 139). Keep the person lying down for better circulation, unless his injuries prohibit it, and keep him warm. The circulatory system may not be able to overcome gravity and get blood to the head if the victim is upright. Elevate the feet 8 to 12 inches to improve circulation, but lower them immediately if the person starts complaining of chest pain or has trouble breathing. If the victim is unconscious or has severe facial injuries, turn him on his side to let blood, vomit or saliva trickle out; otherwise he could choke. Get medical help immediately. If help is more than 2 hours away and the victim isn't vomiting, unconscious or likely to need surgery due to serious injuries, give him fluids. These help replace lost body fluids and increase blood volume to raise blood pressure, which drops so drastically in shock. A solution of baking soda and salt in water works well (see above). If possible, treat the injury that caused the shock.	Treating shock can be enormously complicated by other injuries, so follow the prohibitions for the specific injury. Never move the person if it appears he has head, neck or back injuries. And don't give a shock victim fluids if he's unconscious, in convulsions, vomiting or likely to need surgery because of severe injuries—it complicates the surgeon's job.

Unconsciousness

There are many causes of unconsciousness, and nearly all are *symptoms* of other conditions such as drug overdose, head injury, poisoning, shock, heart attack, heatstroke or electrocution.

Your first task is not to find out what's wrong with an unconscious person, but to save his life. When consciousness is lost, muscles may lose their tone and become floppy. The main danger is suffocation, either because the tongue is blocking the throat or because vomit is stuck there. So be prepared to use artificial respiration (see page 139). And don't leave the victim alone—his breathing could suddenly stop.

How to Check the Pulse

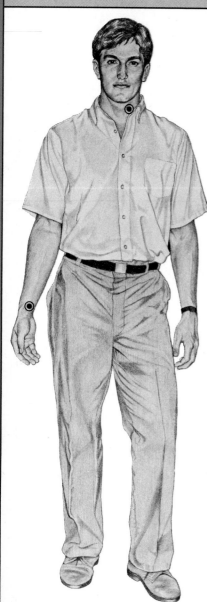

Just as the normal body temperature is 98.6°F, the average normal pulse rate for an adult at rest is 70 beats a minute. (The rate for a newborn baby is 120; for a child, 60 to 90.) Individual pulse rates vary, of course, but if a pulse is significantly above or below these benchmarks, there may be a serious problem.

To find the pulse, place the tips of your second and index fingers on the underside of the person's wrist, just below the thumb. Count the pulsations for 60 seconds. In an infant, check below the left nipple.

If you can't find the pulse on the wrist, or the victim is unconscious, put your fingers into the groove of the neck to either side of the Adam's apple, on the carotid artery, and check there.

When you've done everything you can to help the unconscious person, put him in the recovery position. In this position, the person is prone (face down). The head hangs forward so that the person can breathe freely and liquids can drain easily from the mouth. The bent limbs support the body's weight evenly and comfortably. But *don't* move the person into the recovery position if you suspect a spinal injury, fracture or internal injuries.

1 Make sure clothing is loose and that the victim is breathing; kneel by the person's side.

Recognizing and Treating Fainting

Symptoms and Signs	Action	What Not to Do
Fainting occurs when the blood supply to the brain is reduced for a short time, and recovery follows quickly. Someone about to faint may look very pale, sweat profusely or feel cold to the touch. You can often tell you're going to faint—you feel dizzy and nauseated and have numb or tingling extremities or blurred vision.	The victim almost always regains consciousness when laid down. To prevent a faint, a person feeling weak or dizzy should lie down, or bend over with his head at knee level. If you find someone already passed out, leave him lying down, elevate his feet 8 to 12 inches and loosen any tight clothing. Fainting could signal something far more serious, so keep the victim breathing. If the person starts vomiting, roll him into the recovery position (see below) with his head turned to one side. Check to see if the person has suffered any injuries in falling, then stay with him or have someone else stay while you get medical attention.	Don't pour water on a fainting person's face; it could block his air passages. Instead, bathe his face gently in cold water. Don't give him anything to drink or use smelling salts: They're more a placebo for the rescuer than anything else and could trigger a reaction. If it's just a fainting spell, the person will come out of it without the salts; if it's more serious, salts won't do any good.

The Recovery Position

2 If the victim is on his back, maneuver him into the prone position in this way: Straighten the arm nearest to you and put it above his head. Bend and cross the far arm over the chest, and the far leg over the one nearer you. Grasp the clothing at the hip and pull the person gently over toward you with one hand, rotating the head with the body and protecting the face with the other hand. Be sure the face is resting on the outstretched arm.

3 Draw the near arm from under the body. Bend this arm and the near leg until each one forms an angle with the body, bent at the elbow and knee. Tilt the head back so that the chin juts forward but is lower than the body. Keep the person warm and stay close by to monitor his breathing.

Your Family's Health Diary

Keeping records of your family's health is a good first step in preventive self-care. It will also ensure the best treatment in times of illness. You'll find these pages especially helpful if you change doctors, travel far from home or simply need emergency help. As you record your family's illnesses, you'll notice whether any patterns develop. You'll remember which drug caused an allergic reaction and when it's time for your booster shots. We've even included a home safety checklist to help you keep your household accident free.

You can record information directly on the forms on these pages or use them as models to start your health diary in a separate notebook. Regardless of which method you choose, we recommend that you turn to the last page of this section first and fill in all the emergency numbers right away so you'll have them handy at all times.

Family Health

Family Member	Blood Type	Rh Factor	Height	Weight	Blood Cholesterol Level	Blood Pressure	
						Systolic	Diastolic

Disease History

Family Member	Date of Birth	Date of Death (cause)	Illnesses—at what age/date (include allergies, emotional problems and childhood diseases such as whooping cough, chicken pox, scarlet fever, rheumatic fever)

Immunization Record

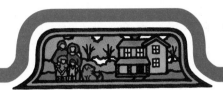

Immunization		Dates				
		Father	Mother	Child	Child	Child
DTP= diphtheria, tetanus, pertussis (whooping cough)	First					
	Second					
	Third					
	Boosters					
Polio	First					
	Second					
	Third					
	Boosters					
Rubella						
Measles						
Mumps						
Smallpox						
Hepatitis B						
Influenza						
Pneumonia						
Tuberculosis (note tests for)						
Other:						

Important Medical Events and Hospitalization Record

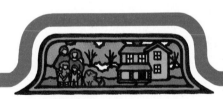

Family Member	Date	Age	What Happened (include complications, length of hospital stay)	Physician

Medications History

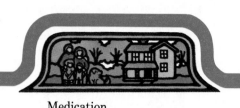

Family Member	Date	Reason for Taking Medication	Medication Used (include strength of dosage)	Problems/ Allergic Reaction	Result/ Comment

Emergency Consent Form

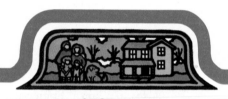

If your child needs emergency medical care and you aren't available to give your formal consent, vital care could be delayed. Leave an up-to-date emergency consent form, like this one, with your emergency telephone numbers list. Whenever you leave your child in another's care, make sure the form is readily accessible. The sitter must bring it to the hospital if emergency care is necessary.

To whom it may concern: In the event of any medical emergency I/we hereby give my/our consent to Dr. _____ or whoever he/she designates to care for our child/children

_____

name(s)

_____

signature

_____

relationship   date

Address and directions to emergency room:

_____
_____
_____
_____

Regional Poison Centers

ARIZONA
Arizona Poison and Drug Information
Center (Tucson)
602-626-6016 (800-362-0101,
Arizona only)

CALIFORNIA
Regional Poison Center,
University of California, Davis
916-453-3692 (800-852-7221,
Northern California only)
San Diego Regional Poison Center
619-294-6000
San Francisco Bay Area Regional
Poison Control Center
415-666-2845 (800-792-0720,
Northern California only)

COLORADO
Rocky Mountain Poison Center (Denver)
303-629-1123 (800-332-3073,
Colorado only)

DISTRICT OF COLUMBIA
National Capitol Poison Center
(Washington, D.C.)
202-625-3333

FLORIDA
Tampa Bay Regional Poison Control
Center
813-251-6995 (800-282-3171,
Florida only)

ILLINOIS
St. John's Hospital Regional Poison
Resource Center (Springfield)
217-753-3330 (800-252-2022,
Illinois only)

INDIANA
Indiana Poison Center (Indianapolis)
317-630-7351 (800-382-9097,
Indiana only)

IOWA
University of Iowa Hospitals and
Clinics Poison Control Center
(Iowa City)
319-356-2922 (800-272-6477,
Iowa only)

KENTUCKY
Kentucky Regional Poison Center of
Kosair-Children's Hospital (Louisville)
502-589-8222 (800-722-5725,
Kentucky only)

MARYLAND
Maryland Poison Center (Baltimore)
301-528-7701 (800-492-2414,
Maryland only)

MASSACHUSETTS
Massachusetts Poison Control System
(Boston)
617-232-2120 (800-682-9211,
Massachusetts only)

MICHIGAN
Children's Hospital of Michigan-South-
east Regional Poison Center (Detroit)
313-494-5711 (800-462-6642;
800-572-1655, Michigan only)

MINNESOTA
Minnesota Poison Control System
St. Paul-Ramsey Medical Center
612-221-2113 (800-222-1222,
Minnesota only)

MISSOURI
Mid-American Poison Center
(Kansas City) 913-588-6633
Cardinal Glennon Memorial Hospital
for Children (St. Louis)
314-772-5200 (800-392-9111,
Missouri only)

NEBRASKA
Mid-Plains Regional Poison Center
(Omaha)
402-390-5400 (800-642-9999,
Nebraska only)

NEW JERSEY
New Jersey Poison Information and
Education System (Newark)
201-926-8005 (800-962-1253,
New Jersey only)

NEW MEXICO
New Mexico Poison, Drug Information
and Medical Crisis Center (Albuquerque)
505-843-2551 (800-432-6866,
New Mexico only)

NEW YORK
Long Island Regional Poison Control
Center (East Meadow)
516-542-2323
New York City Poison Center
212-340-4494
Life Line-Finger Lakes Regional
Poison Control Center (Rochester)
716-275-5151

TEXAS
Southeast Texas Poison Control Center
(Galveston)
409-765-1420; 713-654-1701

UTAH
Inter-Mountain Regional Poison Control
Center (Salt Lake City)
801-581-2151 (800-662-0062,
Utah only)

WASHINGTON
Seattle Poison Center-Children's
Orthopedic Hospital
206-526-2121 (800-732-6985,
Washington only)

Home Safety Checklist

Deaths from accidents in the home rank second in frequency, exceeded only by motor vehicle fatalities. These are all the more tragic because the majority could be prevented by correcting unsafe conditions around the home. Use this checklist to make your home truly safe.

Stairways

- ☐ Stairs well lighted.
- ☐ No objects left to lie on stairways, even temporarily.
- ☐ Carpeting in good condition, with no protruding nails.

Garage, Laundry, Basement, Workshop

- ☐ Keys never left in car ignition. (A child could start the car.)
- ☐ All paints, chemicals, fertilizers and detergents either locked away or stored in their original containers well out of children's reach. When a chemical product is no longer needed, throw it out.
- ☐ Garden tools, power tools well out of reach and disconnected when not in use.
- ☐ Proper ventilation provided when using vaporizing chemicals like turpentine, acetone.
- ☐ Doors removed from old cabinets, refrigerators and freezers.
- ☐ Gas and water lines, fuses and circuit breakers all clearly marked.
- ☐ Flammable substances stored in well-ventilated area, away from heat.
- ☐ Rubbish, oily rags disposed of immediately.
- ☐ Brush or other garden fires never left untended.
- ☐ Ample lighting provided, especially around work areas.

Kitchen

- ☐ Pot handles turned toward the back of the stove to decrease danger of children grabbing them.
- ☐ Household cleaners, detergent stored away from sink, out of children's reach.
- ☐ Plastic bags discarded if not in use.
- ☐ Fire extinguishers kept near stove, fireplace, garage.
- ☐ Knives, all sharp utensils hung up out of reach.
- ☐ Floors covered with a nonslip surface; not overwaxed.
- ☐ Electrical appliances away from sink and stove, unplugged when not in use.
- ☐ Step stool or utility ladder handy for reaching high cupboards and shelves.

Bathroom

- ☐ All drugs, medications and cosmetics either locked up or high out of children's reach. This includes aspirin, cosmetics and shampoo; special attention to razor blades.
- ☐ All medicines clearly labeled. Outdated medicines flushed down the toilet.
- ☐ Nonslip, rubber-bottom mats in the shower, on the floor.
- ☐ Electrical appliances like razors and hair dryers away from sink and tub, unplugged when not in use.

Bedroom

- ☐ Electric blankets unplugged when not in use.
- ☐ Nonflammable bedclothes provided for children.
- ☐ Sleeping pills locked away.
- ☐ Too-soft pillows, blankets removed from small children's bed to decrease danger of suffocation.
- ☐ Lamp or light switch within reach of every bed to prevent falling in the dark; night lights for children.
- ☐ Smoking in bed absolutely prohibited.

General

- ☐ All areas well lighted, especially entrance ways, hallways.
- ☐ Extension cords used only for temporary jobs and removed when job completed.
- ☐ Electrical circuits never overloaded.
- ☐ Electrical cords, stereo cables never under rug and never overextended.
- ☐ Smoke detectors installed.
- ☐ Any guns in the house locked up, with the firing pin removed.
- ☐ Fireplace adequately guarded with screen.
- ☐ Unused electrical outlets covered with heavy electrical tape or plugs.
- ☐ The best escape routes in case of fire rehearsed by all family members.
- ☐ Small children never left unattended.

Emergency Telephone Numbers

Family name and address (include very specific directions for finding residence so emergency vehicles can arrive promptly)

Fire _____

Police _____

Paramedics _____

Hospital
emergency room _____

Regional poison
control center _____

Taxi _____

Gas company _____

Electric company _____

Oil company _____

Water company _____

Dentist _____

     name   office phone   home phone

Pharmacy _____

     name   phone

24-hour pharmacy _____

     name   phone

Father's work phone _____   Mother's work phone _____

Neighbor's phone _____   Relative's phone _____

Family
doctors _____

     name   family member(s) seen   office phone   home phone

     name   family member(s) seen   office phone   home phone

Person to contact
in emergency _____

     name   address   phone

Other numbers _____

Buyer's Guide

Here's where to find the products pictured in this book. Prices are approximate.

Chapter 1

"Self-Care Tools," pages 8-9

Children's stethoscope ($8.50)
The Self-Care Catalog
P.O. Box 999
Point Reyes, CA 94956
415-663-8462

Otoscope with dental mirror ($19.95)
NOTOCO 1983
P.O. Box 300
Ferndale, CA 95536
707-796-4400

Norelco blood pressure kit ($79.95)
Norelco
High Ridge Park
P.O. Box 10166
Stamford, CT 06904
203-329-5700

Vitamin C self-test kit ($10 for 20 tests)
ABROCA, Inc.
P.O. Box 5528
Maple Street Station
Beverly Hills, CA 90210
213-655-9444

Microstix-nitrite test ($2.95 for 3 tests)
Miles Labs
P.O. Box 70
Elkhart, IN 46515
219-264-8645
Also available through
The Self-Care Catalog (see above).

Pregnancy test ($10-$15)
Available at drugstores.

Baby temperature thermometer ($2.69)
Baby Temp
TRP Energy Sensors, Inc.
232 Madison Avenue, Suite 401
New York, NY 10016

Vaginal speculum ($12.95) and basal body thermometer ($6.95)
Available from hospital and medical supply houses and some drugstores, or through *The Self-Care Catalog* (see above).

Emergency dental kit ($20)
Comfortably Yours
52B West Hunter Avenue
Maywood, NJ 07607
201-368-0400

Chapter 2

"Brush Your Headache Away," page 12
Classic British Bath Brush ($25-$55)
Caswell-Massey Co.
111 Eighth Avenue
New York, NY 10011
212-620-0900

Reversible Blanket Support ($20), page 26
Comfortabiy Yours
52B West Hunter Avenue
Maywood, NJ 07607
201-368-0400

"Just Hangin' Around," page 32
Orthopod ($300)
Brilhante Co., Inc.
3283 Motor Avenue
West Los Angeles, CA 90034
213-559-6900
800-821-6275 (in California)

"Tools That Work to Save Your Back," pages 38-39

Items are available through the Comfortably Yours catalog,
52B West Hunter Ave.,
Maywood, NJ 07607,
201-368-0400,
unless otherwise noted.

Backsaver Shovel ($24.50)

Backsaver Rake ($15.50)

Balans Chair ($200-$325)
Hag U.S. Importers
Room 1052, Merchandise Mart
Chicago, IL 60654
312-222-0166

Neck support ($16.50)

Adjustable back support ($32)

Long Reach Washer ($42)

Lawn Claws ($34.50)

Moist heat heating pad ($57)

Source Notes

Chapter 1

Page 2

"The Rising Cost of Disease" adapted from *1981-1982 Source Book of Health Insurance Data,* by the Health Insurance Association of America (Washington, D.C.: Health Insurance Association of America, 1982).

Page 6

"Side Effects of 'Safe' Drugs" adapted from *Handbook of Nonprescription Drugs,* 7th ed., by the American Pharmaceutical Association (Washington, D.C.: American Pharmaceutical Association, 1982) and *Physicians' Desk Reference for Nonprescription Drugs,* 4th ed., Barbara B. Huff, ed. (Oradell, N.J.: Medical Economics, 1983) and *The Merck Manual,* 14th ed., by Robert Berkow, M.D. (Rahway, N.J.: Merck & Co., 1982). and *Physicians' Desk Reference,* 38th ed., (Oradell, N.J.: Medical Economics, 1984) and *The People's Pharmacy -2* by Joe Graedon with Teresa Graedon (New York: Avon Books, 1980) and *Dr. Fishbein's Popular Illustrated Medical Encyclopedia,* by Morris Fishbein, M.D. (Garden City, N.Y.: Doubleday, 1979).

Chapter 3

Pages 50-51

"A Guide to Diagnosis, Self-Care and Medical Treatment" adapted from *Healthy Sex and Keeping It That Way,* by Richard Lumiere, M.D., and Stephani Cook (New York: Simon & Schuster, 1983) and "How to Deal with Sexually Transmitted Diseases," by Michael Castleman, *Medical Self-Care,* Spring 1983 and

The American Medical Association Family Medical Guide, Jeffrey R. M. Kunz, M.D., ed. (New York: Random House, 1982) and *Better Homes and Gardens New Family Medical Guide,* Edwin Kiester, Jr., ed. (Des Moines: Meredith, 1982) and *Take Care of Yourself,* by Donald Vickery, M.D., and James Fries, M.D. (Reading, Mass.: Addison-Wesley, 1981) and *Medical Self-Care and Assessment,* by Brent Q. Hafen, Ph.D. (Englewood, Colo.: Morton, 1983).

Chapter 4

Page 62

"Are You Burned Out?" adapted from a chart, "Burnout Syndrome," compiled by Shobhana V. Vora, M.D., of the Mission Viejo Medical Center, Mission Viejo, Calif.

Chapter 8

Page 127

"Alkaline-Acid Effects of Some Common Foods." This information is adapted from *Hawk's Physiological Chemistry* (McGraw-Hill, Inc., 1965). All foods are calculated in the raw state and are meant as a guide for estimating average portions or servings.

Chapter 9

Pages 133-161

"Emergency First Aid" adapted from *Standard First Aid and Personal Safety,* by the American Red Cross (Garden City, N.Y.: Doubleday, 1979) and *The American Medical Association's Handbook of First Aid and Emergency Care,* by the American Medical Association (New York: Random House, 1980.) and *Dr. Heimlich's Home Guide to Emergency Medical Situations,* by Henry J. Heimlich, M.D., with Lawrence Galton (New York: Simon & Schuster, 1980)

Page 150

"Meet Mr. Yuk." "Mr. Yuk" sticker reproduced by permission of the Institute of Education Communications, Children's Hospital of Pittsburgh, 125 DeSoto Street, Pittsburgh, PA 15213

Photography Credits

Cover: Sally Shenk Ullman.
Staff Photographers— Christopher Barone: pp. 5; 8-9; 40-41; 64; 108; 109; 111, bottom right; 113, bottom left; 122, center and bottom right; 126, top left; 128; 132-133. Angelo M. Caggiano: pp. 10-11; 30-31; 43; 75; 130, center. Carl Doney: pp. viii-1; 96-97; 120, bottom right; 124, top left; 130, top left. T. L. Gettings: pp. 82-83; 114, top right; 124, bottom left. John P. Hamel: pp. 100, top right; 116, bottom left. Mark Lenny: pp. 52; 56-57. Mitchell T. Mandel: pp. 16; 32; 34-35; 58-59; 66, bottom right; 95; 101; 112, bottom left; 121, top right; 127. Alison Miksch: pp. 23; 26; 104; 106; 107. Anthony Rodale: pp. 12, center; 25; 44. Margaret Skrovanek: pp. 7; 15, top; 37; 63; 69; 73; 76; 77; 110-111; 113, top right; 115; 116, top left; 118; 119; 122, top left; 123, top right; 125, bottom left. Christie C. Tito: pp. 12, bottom; 15, bottom; 18-19; 38-39; 66, bottom left; 112, top right; 125, top; 131, center. Sally Shenk Ullman: pp. 117; 121, bottom right. Rodale Press Photography Department: pp. 114, center; 120, top right; 124, center; 130, bottom left; 131, top.

Other Photographers— Mario Ruiz/Picture Group: p. 28. Donna Kruetz: p. 55. Four by Five/Bob Hewellyn: p. 86. Tony Barboza: pg. 100, bottom left. Jane C. Knutila: p. 121, center. Steve Marx: p. 129.

Additional Photographs Courtesy of— A. Devaney, Inc.: p. 87. Charles C. Roberts, Jr.: p. 94.

Illustration Credits

Bascove: pp. 20-21; 44-45; 81; 105; 156; 157; 158; 160. Susan Blubaugh: pp. 61; 90; 98-99; 102-103. Jerry O'Brien: pp. 72; 125. Mary Anne Shea: pp. 2; 6; 23; 33; 84; 85; 88; 89; 112; 113; 114; 115; 116; 117; 118; 119; 120; 123; 125, top; 126; 127; 129; 131. Elwood Smith: pp. 70-71. Chris Spollen: pp. 4; 65; 68; 93. Wendy Wray: pp. 134; 135; 136; 138; 139; 141; 142; 143; 144; 146; 147; 148; 154; 155.

Special thanks to— Bamberger's, Whitehall, Pa.; Nazareth Sporting Goods, Nazareth, Pa.; Nestor's Sporting Goods, Whitehall, Pa.; Que-ma-ho-ning Indian Post, Allentown, Pa.; Mrs. J. I. Rodale, Allentown, Pa.; Van B's Pony Farm, Nazareth, Pa.; Brent Whitehead, New Jersey Regional Poison Control Center, Newark, N.J.

Index

U

Ulcers
    cabbage and, 103
    skin, benefits of wine for, 125
Ultraviolet rays, protection from, 93-94
Unconsciousness, 154-55
Urethritis, 50-51, 53
Urinary tract infections, cranberry
    juice for, 102
Urine, acidic, smoking and, 127
Uva ursi, 99

V

Vaginal infections, 50-51, 105
Valsalva's maneuver, 22
Vaporizer, 119
Varicose veins, 78-79
Vascular headaches, 13
Venereal disease. *See* Sexually transmit-
    ted diseases (STDs)
Venous bleeding, 134
Vinegar, 105
Vitamin A, 46, 76, 77

Vitamin B_1, as insect repellent, 91
Vitamin B_6
    deficiency of, MSG sensitivity
        and, 115
    for menstrual cramps, 29
Vitamin B_{12}, 60
Vitamin C
    benefits of, 43, 46, 60, 92
    chewable, teeth and, 122
    sources of, 60
Vitamin E, 27, 49, 76, 105
Vitamins
    hangover and, 65
    best time to take, 130

W

Waking up, exercises for, 58-59
Walking, benefits of, 27, 28, 78
Warts, garlic for, 103
Washing, effect of on skin, 120
Water retention, reducing, 128
Water-soluble vitamins, 130

Weight loss, 115, 121
Wine
    calories in, 121
    for skin ulcers, 125
Workaholic boss, how to handle, 63
Workshop, safety checklist for, 160
Worldwide Health Forecast, 124
Wounds
    bandages for, 128
    treatment of, 105

Y

Yeast infections, 50-51, 105
Yellow dock, for itching, 105
Yoga, for menstrual cramps, 29

Z

Zinc
    for colds, 46-47
    for acne, 77
Zinc sulfate, for cold sores, 49
Zori, benefits of for feet, 24-25